The Essential Guide
to Becoming a Doctor

The Essential Guide to Becoming a Doctor

THIRD EDITION

Adrian Blundell
BMedSci, BM, BS, MRCP, MMedSci, MAcad MEd
Consultant,
Health Care of the Elderly and General Medicine,
Nottingham University Hospitals NHS Trust, UK

Richard Harrison
BMedSci, BM, BS, MRCS, MD, MRCGP
General Practitioner
Windsor

Benjamin Turney
MA MB BChir MSc DPhil MRCS PGDipLATHE
Clinical Lecturer in Urology,
Nuffield Department of Surgery,
University of Oxford

Cartoons by

Rebecca Herbertson
BMedSci, BM, BS, MRCP, MSc, DM
Medical Oncology SpR
Sussex Cancer Centre
Brighton and Sussex University Hospitals NHS Trust

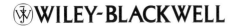

WILEY-BLACKWELL

BMJ|Books

A John Wiley & Sons, Ltd., Publication

This edition first published 2011, © 2004 (BMJ Publishing Group), 2007, 2011 by Adrian Blundell, Richard Harrison and Benjamin Turney

BMJ Books is an imprint of BMJ Publishing Group Limited, used under licence by Blackwell Publishing which was acquired by John Wiley & Sons in February 2007. Blackwell's publishing programme has been merged with Wiley's global Scientific, Technical and Medical business to form Wiley-Blackwell.

Registered office: John Wiley & Sons Ltd, The Atrium, Southern Gate, Chichester, West Sussex, PO19 8SQ, UK

Editorial offices: 9600 Garsington Road, Oxford, OX4 2DQ, UK

 The Atrium, Southern Gate, Chichester, West Sussex, PO19 8SQ, UK

 111 River Street, Hoboken, NJ 07030-5774, USA

For details of our global editorial offices, for customer services and for information about how to apply for permission to reuse the copyright material in this book please see our website at www.wiley.com/wiley-blackwell

Library of Congress Cataloging-in-Publication Data

Blundell, Adrian.
The essential guide to becoming a doctor / Adrian Blundell, Richard Harrison, Benjamin Turney ; cartoons by Rebecca Herbertson. — 3rd ed.
 p. ; cm.
 Includes index.
 ISBN 978-0-470-65455-2
 1. Medicine—Great Britain—Vocational guidance. I. Harrison, Richard.
 II. Turney, Benjamin. III. Title.
[DNLM: 1. Medicine—Great Britain—Popular Works. 2. Career Choice—Great Britain—Popular Works. 3. Education, Medical—Great Britain—Popular Works. 4. Vocational Guidance—Great Britain—Popular Works. W 21 B658e 2011]
 R690.B64 2011
 610.69—dc22
 2010024517

A catalogue record for this book is available from the British Library.

This book is published in the following electronic formats: ePDF 9781444329759; Wiley Online Library 9781444329742; ePub 9781444329766

Set in 9.5/12 pt Minion by MPS Limited, a Macmillan Company, Chennai, India
Printed and bound in Singapore by Fabulous Printers Pte Ltd

1   2011

Contents

Preface to the first edition

So you want to be a doctor? Have you asked yourself why?

Doctors have a highly privileged role. Medics are involved in peoples' lives from facilitating their conception to dignifying their death. Medicine can be a rewarding career despite constant concerns regarding hours, pay, and working conditions. Consequently, competition for places at medical school is high and on the increase.

Deciding to choose medicine is a decision that has lifelong and lifestyle implications. Do you know that you will have to spend 5 years at university and then up to 15 years before reaching the top of your profession? Do you know what being on call means? Even more importantly do you have any idea what life at university and a career as a doctor will be like?

Look no further because help is at hand. Here is the completely unbiased, honest, and unadulterated guide to telling you everything you ever wanted to know about being a doctor – and a lot more. From the initial application right through to training in your chosen speciality – it's all here.

We have written this book to help you make a decision about a career in medicine. We hope that you find it helpful. Personally we had little or no idea what we were letting ourselves in for. Lucky for us it was the right decision and we love it. Sadly for some it isn't. Careful thought early on should prevent this; remember there are other rewarding careers.

Life at university is fantastic, no arguments. Life as a doctor has great moments, but be under no illusion, it is hard work, at times routine, and it can be stressful. Read this book and embark on your career with your eyes and ears open. Work hard but more importantly remember to take time to play hard.

Please remember that courses and application procedures change, as can working patterns and practices. It is advisable to check the latest information before applying.

Good luck!
Adrian Blundell
Richard Harrison
Benjamin Turney
2004

Preface to the third edition

Despite the growing number of places available for medical students, universities are expecting more and more from applicants. Required A-level grades are becoming higher, admission tests have been introduced and a greater emphasis than ever before is being placed on extracurricular activities and work experience. Training as a medical student and life as a doctor has changed considerably since the first edition of this book, nearly ten years ago. The idea of being a doctor can be very different to the reality. Do your research, and plenty of it; if you still want to become a doctor, then go for it – there are few more rewarding careers for those who choose wisely.

Our reasons for writing this book have not changed and our general advice hasn't either. However many of the specifics are continually changing and will continue to do so with the recent change of government. It is essential to keep up to date, even at an early stage of your career.

We wish you every success in your future career, whatever you choose.

Adrian Blundell
Richard Harrison
Benjamin Turney
2011

Acknowledgements

We are extremely grateful to the following people for their contributions and comments:

Julian Boullin Specialist Registrar in Cardiology, Southampton University Hospitals NHS Trust

Tim Brabants Specialty Registrar, Acute Medicine, Nottingham University Hospitals NHS Trust

Eleanor Dittner Foundation Year 1 Doctor, Nottingham University Hospitals NHS Trust

Torquil Duncan-Brown General Practitioner, Litchfield

Bryony Elliott Specialty Registrar, Sherwood Hospitals NHS Foundation Trust

Alice Gallen Final Year Medical Student, University College London

Alex Glover Foundation Year 2 Doctor, Nottingham University Hospitals NHS Trust

Adam Gordon Clinical Lecturer in Medicine of Older People, Division of Rehabilitation and Ageing, University of Nottingham

Rebecca Herbertson Specialist Registrar in Medical Oncology, Brighton and Sussex University Hospitals NHS Trust

James Hopkinson General Practitioner, Nottingham

Emma Lane Foundation Year 2 Doctor, Palmerston North, New Zealand

John MacFarlane Consultant Physician and Professor of Respiratory Medicine, Nottingham University Hospitals NHS Trust

Sir Peter Morris Former President of the Royal College of Surgeons of England

Pip Parson	Foundation Year 2 Doctor, Royal Derby Hospitals NHS Foundation Trust
David Powis	Assistant Dean and Director of Teaching and Learning University of Newcastle, Australia
Zudin Puthucheary	Clinical lecturer in intensive care, Institute of health and human performance University College, London
Jamie Read	5th Year Medical Student, Peninsula Medical School
Anna Rich	Specialist Registrar, Respiratory Medicine, Nottingham University Hospitals NHS Trust
Jeremy Snape	Consultant Physician, Sherwood Forest Hospitals NHS Foundation Trust
Gemma Wilkinson	General Practitioner, Nottingham

Chapter 1 **A challenging career**

1.1 Medicine or not

The decision to study medicine at university should not be made without a great deal of thought and research into the reality of life as a doctor. At the age of 17 it can be difficult to know whether you want to go to university at all, let alone study for at least 5 years. Your future career ideas should be discussed with family and friends but the final decision needs to be an individual one. Those around you are likely to have differing views; parents and teachers may feel that medicine is a respected profession and possibly encourage you to take this path but some doctors may try to dissuade you. Speak to as many students, doctors and other healthcare professionals as possible in order to gain as many opinions as possible. Ask individuals to justify their reasoning for choosing medicine as a career and to explain why they would or would not recommend it; without experiencing life as a doctor, it is difficult to know what it will really be like. We all know friends who have avoided medicine following their personal experience with one or both parents as doctors. In comparison many students, after experiencing their own family life, do decide to follow in their parents' footsteps. Although relatively common, try not to be persuaded or coerced into studying medicine by your family – it is YOUR decision and YOUR career for the rest of your life.

For older candidates, the decision is even more difficult. A mature student needs to be certain that the decision to study medicine is the right one as often there is more at stake; each applicant will have their own personal circumstances but returning to student life may involve leaving paid employment and moving a family around the country.

1.2 Career planning portfolio

A useful starting point on the application pathway is to buy a scrapbook or folder for developing into a useful resource full of ideas and information. Early

The Essential Guide to Becoming a Doctor, 3rd edition. © Adrian Blundell, Richard Harrison and Benjamin Turney. Published 2011 by Blackwell Publishing Ltd.

pages should be dedicated to listing your possible career or degree choices. For each decision produce a table with two columns headed 'Advantages' and 'Disadvantages'.

Possible advantages of a career in medicine

- Five years at university
- Interesting
- Virtual guarantee of job following graduation
- Reasonable salary
- Respected profession
- Diverse range of specialties
- Option to use both intellectual and technical abilities
- Continual advances in the profession
- Sociable work environment
- Good team-working opportunities
- Managerial and leadership opportunities
- Structured career
- Transferable skills
- Opportunities for working abroad

If you find the disadvantages column dominating at any point, then think carefully whether this decision is correct. Portfolios are used extensively in the medical profession, from medical students to senior doctors, as a record of training that can be used as evidence of competence (i.e. the ability to carry out one's job). Your portfolio can be divided into different sections: academic; work experience diary; extracurricular activities; employment; managerial, leadership and organizational skills; university choices; commitment to medicine (or other degree); newspaper/journal articles; curriculum vitae. Rather than just listing achievements, it is sensible to reflect on your experiences, for example what were the good and bad bits and how they have helped towards your future career choice. This will develop into an essential resource that will aid your future career choice decision and will be useful to look through prior to interviews.

Possible disadvantages of a career in medicine

- Five years at university
- Long hours
- Lots of exams
- Risk of mistakes

- Stressful periods
- Dealing with death/suffering
- Patient expectations
- Media bashing
- Paperwork
- Lack of NHS funding
- Possible job insecurity
- Lack of flexibility in training
- Litigation (being sued)

1.3 The decision

University is only the tip of the medical career iceberg; the remaining 40 years of medicine can be quite different. There is no doubt that a career as a doctor can be challenging, rewarding and exciting, but remember that it is also hard work, stressful, tiring and, at times, mundane. Have you the right personality, not just for the university course but also in the longer term? The majority of sixth form students have no idea what university and a career in medicine will be like, and embark on this journey blinkered by this lack of insight. However, knowledge can be gained by talking to current medical students, career advisors, general practitioners, hospital doctors, and by reading books on the topic of studying medicine and perusing the medical journals. It is also necessary to spend time in and around a hospital or GP surgery, known as work experience or voluntary work. This is an essential prerequisite for obtaining a place at medical school as it shows your commitment, but it is also necessary for gaining more insight into your future career choice.

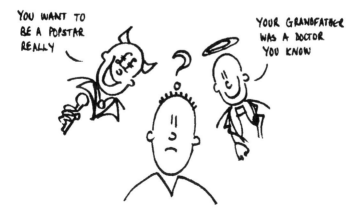

The decision to study medicine at university should not be made without a great deal of thought

Students have differing motivations for choosing a medical career: family tradition has been discussed, others have experienced medicine as a patient, some have an interest in science, a minority have wanted to become a doctor since the dawn of time, and many just feel that they want to help people. Having experienced medicine from the point of view of being a patient or relative is useful and these experiences can be shared on application forms or at interview. Some of your friends may well know that it is their destiny to become a brain surgeon but the odds are that these people will change their minds over the forthcoming years. The idea of a specialty is different to the reality. It is not necessary for you to decide on your future career prior to applying to medical school, but if you do have some thoughts then these can be mentioned, although remember to have reasons to justify your decision. For many the final decision to study medicine will be made shortly before sending off the UCAS form. Whatever your reason for thinking medicine is your future, it is important to realize that there are other jobs and university courses that would fulfil these reasons and a life following one of these different paths could be just as rewarding. Remember that there are a number of wrong reasons for pursuing medicine as a career.

While deciding on a medical career, it is important not to be disillusioned by the negative media publicity or the drama depicted in television programmes; these are two ends of an extensive spectrum and the majority of the work of a doctor is different. In terms of adverse publicity, remember that doctors have not just started to make mistakes, that doctors probably make fewer mistakes now than ever before, and that the difference is due to the expectation and knowledge of the general public. Mistakes are now less tolerated, and with the advent of the internet patients are more aware of their diseases and also of treatment options.

If you are serious about studying to become a doctor, in addition to researching about life as a doctor (including quality work experience), it is necessary to determine that you have the right attributes and qualities. Although academic excellence does not always equate to good clinical skills as a doctor, there are minimum requirements for entry into medical school. If you have performed badly in your GCSEs or are not likely to get high grades at A level, it is unlikely that you will be offered a place to study medicine, as there is great competition. A useful starting point is to look at the UCAS website for the minimum requirements for entry to each university. Apart from academic pursuits, it is important that applicants demonstrate other interests and abilities and most candidates will have a history of sporting or musical interests and be able to demonstrate leadership and team-working experiences. All these attributes are important for a future healthcare professional, and universities are looking for well-rounded individuals.

There may be other options available if exam results are disappointing at AS level and predicted A-level grades lower than required, and some of these options are discussed in later chapters. Possibilities to consider include resitting A levels and studying a different degree at university and then applying for graduate-entry medicine at a later date. The key is getting excellent A-level grades – if you have the academic requirements for a university place, and the suitable attributes and qualities of a future doctor, then you should be able to get an interview offer, even if this means taking a year off to reapply.

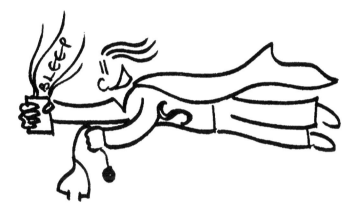

The job of a doctor can be challenging, rewarding, exciting . . .

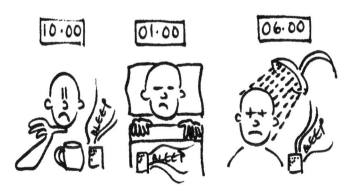

. . . but also hard work, stressful, boring and routine

The decision to study medicine is just the beginning. Now it is necessary to decide which university and, for some students, which country. It is likely you will have a great time at whichever institution you find yourself. Remember that not all universities are the same and at some the workload could be greater and the social life less. This is why research before applying could save heartache later. Once at medical school, the majority of those students who wish to become doctors do eventually make it through. Some decide that medicine is not the career for them and either leave or convert to another degree. Likewise, some students embark on other science degrees and find that medicine would be more suitable, so make the change then. If you are unsure about your future career, then a possible option might be to study at a medical school offering intercalated degrees as part of the course. For example, at Nottingham the preclinical work includes a research project in the third year that leads to the degree of Bachelor of Medical Science (BMedSci); after this a student could leave the medical school and pursue an alternative career with a degree under his or her belt.

1.4 A changing profession

Medical training and the health service have undergone radical changes in the last 5 years. It is unusual for a day to go by without some mention in the press about changes in doctor training and cuts having to be made due to financial problems. The main push is for a quality health service at an affordable price. Morale has been low due to hospital closures and job uncertainty for many healthcare professionals. It is essential as potential future doctors that even at this early stage you stay up to date with the proposed alterations to career structure, training and NHS reforms. Although it may seem irrelevant at your stage in life, the changes may well alter your decision to study medicine. One interesting aspect is that with the increased number of places at medical school and the reduction in the number of training posts, we may see unemployed doctors for the first time. Employment following graduation is virtually guaranteed but greater competition during later training may mean limited possibilities, especially in smaller specialties and popular locations. Modernizing Medical Careers (MMC) is a government-led initiative that was introduced in 2007 to make training at all levels more formalized. Following medical school, newly qualified doctors now join a 2-year Foundation programme rather than the traditional 1-year Pre-registration House Officer (previously known as the Junior House Officer year). More information about current and future training can be found in later chapters.

1.5 Planning

Planning and research are the key components in deciding and then ultimately applying for medicine. Try to prepare well in advance. Here is a checklist to help formulate a few ideas, although it is by no means exhaustive.

Choosing a medical career: a planning checklist

- *Keep a scrapbook or folder*: develop a plan for a medical career, divided into sections as described earlier. Remember to keep informative newspaper cuttings or journal articles and to write about your experiences rather than just listing achievements.
- *Academia*: at an early stage determine which subjects you need at AS and A2 level. Work hard to obtain the required marks! As well as your A-level work, consider some general reading around medical topics. *Nature* and the *British Medical Journal* are good starting points; the *BMJ* is one of the most widely read journals in medicine and the student version has useful articles on career planning and changes in training and also presents interesting medical cases. At a minimum you should be aware of medical advances and developments that have made the lay press and look at these in more detail.
- *Requirements*: a good starting point is the UCAS website (www.ucas.org); this has information on the necessary requirements for every course at UK universities. It also has a careers advice questionnaire program that can map your interests and abilities to potential careers and also lots of other general information for potential students. If you are required to pass an extra exam prior to applying (e.g. UKCAT), then make sure you submit applications for these (see Chapter 3).
- *General Medical Council* (www.gmc-uk.org): the GMC is the regulatory body for doctors. It produces multiple publications with information for doctors. A useful start would be to look through the booklets *Good Medical Practice* and *Tomorrows Doctors*.
- *Department of Health* (www.dh.gov.uk): keep abreast of developments in the health service by looking at the Department of Health website. Find summary documents on important governmental papers and legislation.
- *Modernizing Medical Careers* (www.mmc.nhs.uk): look through the recent developments in medical training.
- *Research your future career*: speak to as many doctors (community and hospital), medical students and other healthcare professionals as you can.
- *Work experience*: you need to be organized to sort this in good time. The quality is more important than the quantity and consider a variety of experiences.
- *Medical school research*: request the prospectus from the universities you are considering applying to and look at their websites. Make sure you attend the university open days and take the opportunity to speak to as many students as possible and look around the town or surrounding areas (see Chapter 5).
- *Extracurricular activities*: as with work experience, it is about the skills and attributes you have gained from your interests outside academia rather than merely the number of hobbies you have.

- *'Premedics' groups*: rather than isolating yourself from your peers, why not start a small group of students interested in doing medicine to share ideas, knowledge and experiences.
- *Referee*: start planning in advance who your referee will be. Ensure that he or she has been aware of your commitment to medicine and also that they are fully supportive of your application.
- *Interview practice*: once you have offers, or even earlier if possible, organize mock interviews with several teachers. Practice asking and answering interview questions in your 'premedic' group.

1.6 Summary

There is no one good or bad reason for studying (or not) to become a doctor. It should be a decision that a student is completely happy with and should not be made lightly. For many, a career as a doctor is usually enjoyable and rewarding, but there are times when it can interfere with personal and family life and this can be seen in the higher rate of divorce, depression, alcohol problems and suicide among medical practitioners. With the changes in working practice and the reduction in hours, the impact on personal life should reduce. To help make your chosen career less stressful, it is important not to bottle up emotions but to talk through any problems with friends and colleagues and to have other interests outside medicine in order to relax.

PERSONAL VIEW *Adrian Blundell*

I do not remember when I decided to become a doctor; my first career ambition was to become a pilot, but my early enthusiasm was not shared by my parents. They felt being a pilot would not allow a favourable work/life balance due to the long hours and the frequent trips abroad. My parents are not from a medical background and so possibly didn't realize the long hours involved in being a doctor. Nevertheless, the idea of being a fast jet pilot was then out of my head. At school, I was fairly good at science and reasonable at the arts. The headache initially was deciding my A levels: science and study medicine, or arts and study law. (This limitation in my choice reflected my naivety about the possible careers available and also a rather disappointing lack of careers advice at school.) Science it was and medicine followed.

My teachers were not particularly generous when predicting my A-level grades (BBC). This was actually fair, as my results in the lower sixth form exams were quite poor. The most common offer in 1990 when I was applying to medical school was BBB, and for this reason I ended up obtaining only one offer from a London college. Other universities I applied to wrote back with offers for other degree courses but I had decided on medicine and turned these down. I actually contacted the medical schools to ask why they had not offered me a place – one response was that I had not done any voluntary work. This might have been true at the time of applying but I spent a large majority of my upper sixth helping at the local hospital.

Results day arrived; I had achieved BBB. A difficult decision ensued as I had obtained the necessary grades to take my medical school place, but I was uncertain as to whether I wanted to spend the next 5 years in London. I really wanted to go to a university rather than a medical school so I declined the London offer, and took a gap year. I then had to commence the application procedure once more.

I was unsure exactly what to do with this year. I had no guarantees of getting an offer and would not find out for several months. An advert appeared in the local paper for a school-leaver with science A levels to work in the field of cancer research at a local pharmaceutical company. I successfully applied for this position and then began the process of reapplication to medical school. Many of my friends spent their year jet-setting around the world. Although a little envious, I still had the problem of finding a place at medical school and this prevented me from leaving the country for long stretches. On this occasion I applied to the University of Nottingham, as I had studied the prospectus and liked the idea of a more modern course. I had never even visited the city before, but on the day of my interview I had a gut feeling that this was the place I really wanted to spend my university days. Fortunately, an offer appeared through my door 2 weeks later. The rest, as they say, is history.

During a gap year, the choices include work, travel, or stay around your home town living off your parents' generosity. The latter is to be avoided and universities will not look favourably at this. Work or travel is the main question. Most students undertake a bit of both. From personal experience this is probably the best advice, although working for the whole year did mean that I had some beer money when I left for university and also a car in which to carry it. The decision is yours! Good luck.

Chapter 2 **The application procedure**

2.1 General advice

All applications to university or college courses have to be directed through the University and Colleges Admission Service (UCAS). All applications are now completed online as paper forms no longer exist.

Initially, the task of completing the UCAS application can be quite daunting; after all, this will essentially determine whether you obtain an interview offer and subsequently a university place to study medicine. Do not lose heart: everything in this book is designed to allow you to make an informed decision about your future career, and this chapter guides you stepwise through the application procedure. We will give you hints and tips as to how to complete the form, tell you exactly how the UCAS application system works, and guide you through the application step by step.

Medicine is one of the most popular subjects chosen by undergraduates, and is also one of the most competitive. To be accepted to study medicine, candidates need high grades at A level (or equivalent qualifications), a strong interest in the medical profession and good 'people skills'. Medicine is a profession that combines an intellectual challenge with a strong sense of vocation and contact with a wide range of people.

2.2 Timing your application

Application dates

Application dates differ according to your chosen course and, in the case of medicine, are earlier. For the majority of subjects, your UCAS application must be submitted before mid-January of the year in which you wish to enter university. For medicine, however, you must apply 3 months before this, by mid-October (usually 15 October). Candidates applying for medicine

The Essential Guide to Becoming a Doctor, 3rd edition. © Adrian Blundell,
Richard Harrison and Benjamin Turney. Published 2011 by Blackwell Publishing Ltd.

are not entirely alone in having to apply early; those wishing to apply for any course at Oxford or Cambridge, and those applying for dentistry or veterinary medicine, must also apply early.

Late applications

UCAS state that 'the universities and colleges guarantee to consider your application if we receive your application by the appropriate deadline'; in other words, if your application is received after the deadline date, they may consider it but there is no obligation for them to do so. Our advice would be to never apply after this deadline without extenuating circumstances. The competition for places is high, so any reason to reject your application will be taken, and a late application is certainly high up on this list. Give yourself the best chance – apply as early as possible.

Deferred entry to university

The subject of deferred entry, also known as a gap year, is considered in more detail in Chapter 4. If you are considering taking deferred entry, you must first check that the university or college will actually accept a deferred entry application. When applying for deferred entry, you must obviously meet the same conditions of offer as those not taking a year out. If you accept a place for deferred entry, you cannot reapply through UCAS in the subsequent year unless you withdraw your original application.

If you do want to defer entry to university for a year, it is not compulsory to apply to UCAS during your A-level year, as you can apply during the gap year. This can be useful if you are unsure of what you really want to study, or if your exam results do not meet expectations. However, if considering a delayed application, we recommend that you talk this over with your teachers and career advisers.

2.3 The application process

There are those who seem to know they were born to enter the medical profession, but many doctors, most of them excellent and dedicated, were not sure which career to follow until the night before the UCAS application deadline! The best advice is to find out as much as you can about medicine and the different medical schools before you complete your application. You can do this by reading university prospectuses, speaking to your careers adviser and visiting the university or college. Talk to your family and friends, particularly those who have been to the universities or colleges that you are considering. It might also be wise to attend one of the available conferences held for 16–18 year olds interested in a career as a doctor. These are held in various locations around the country several times a year and usually involve presentations by medical students and doctors of all levels from junior to professor. Many of them hold practical sessions and small group tutorials. The main aim is to give advice on the application process and to give a feel for what a future career as a doctor may be like. Although attending one of these courses does not guarantee an offer of a place at medical school, it does show a commitment to finding out about your possible career choice. You should be happy with your choice of course and university before you make your final decision. Remember, you will be spending the next 5 or 6 years there!

All applications need to be made using the UCAS secure online application system, APPLY. More detailed information can be found at www.ucas .ac.uk. APPLY can be accessed from any computer with an internet connection. Most students will make their application through a school or college and in these cases it is necessary to obtain the individual school's log in. It is also possible for individuals to apply. The application can be changed at any time (until submitted) and we would advise printing it out to check before sending. Once complete and you are satisfied with the content, the application is submitted to UCAS through a school staff member who will add your reference. Individual applicants will need to register themselves for APPLY and also sort out their own references and include these before submitting the form. Applicants can pay online or the school can be invoiced.

When you do apply, remember to print out or save copies of the whole application for your own records and check thoroughly before submitting. Always review a copy before any university interviews.

2.4 Completing the UCAS application step by step

Registration
You need to register to use APPLY; you enter personal details, such as your name, address and date of birth. The registration process generates your username and you create your own password, which you use to log in to APPLY.

Personal details
This section is populated from the registration section above. Most of this information is used to uniquely identify you and to help in the carefully maintained UCAS demographics. You are also asked about any disabilities you may have.

Additional information
You are then asked for information about any non-examination-based activities you have undertaken in preparation for higher education (e.g. summer schools), together with other information designed to help the universities

and colleges to monitor applications in terms of equal opportunities, such as your national identity and ethnic origin.

Choices

In this section you enter the courses, universities and colleges that you are applying to. You can choose up to five courses, which APPLY will arrange into alphabetical order. The order of your choices does not indicate any preference – your application will be sent to all chosen universities and colleges at the same time. Each university and college will only see details of the particular course or courses for which you have applied. They will not see your other choices until you have received your final decision.

You can apply to a maximum of:
- four courses in any one of medicine, dentistry, veterinary medicine or veterinary science;
- one course at either the University of Oxford or the University of Cambridge.

You can use your remaining choice for any other subject. For example, if you have made four choices for medicine, you could still make one choice for dentistry or another subject if you wished. However, you should bear in mind that your personal statement, which often contains course-biased information, will be sent to all the universities and colleges you have chosen.

Another important point when applying for medicine is that when you start your medical training, you will be immunized against hepatitis B. Some universities ask for proof (certificate) that you are not infected with hepatitis B. If you think there is a possibility that you may be infected, you should check directly with the university.

In order to complete this section, it is necessary to know the code names for both the universities and the courses. These are summarized at the end of this chapter.

Education

You then enter where you have studied and which qualifications you are taking or have taken.

Which qualifications should be included?

The simple answer is: *all* your qualifications. It is likely that you have completed GCSEs and AS levels, and these are the first to enter here, but any of the following should be included.
- AS levels
- GCSEs
- Intermediate GNVQs (General National Vocational Qualifications)
- Key skills
- Royal School of Music (RSM) qualifications.

In this section you are trying to convince people that:
- you have the aptitude for medicine;
- you also have other, non-academic interests.

What qualifications do I need to be considered for medical school?
The academic standards necessary for medical school are generally quite high, but there is a small degree of interuniversity variability. *Three* GCEs at advanced (A) level (one usually being Chemistry), or the equivalent level in the Scottish Qualifications Certificate, are the normal *minimum* entry qualifications for medicine. However, in practice you should have *three* A levels with good grades (A and B grades in most cases). These should normally be taken in one single sitting. All medical schools accept a combination of A levels and AS levels. Candidates with the Scottish Certificate intending to apply to universities outside Scotland should check the entry qualifications with each university.

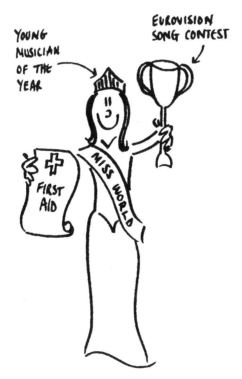

What qualifications do I need to be considered for medical school?

All medical schools usually insist that candidates have an A or AS level in Chemistry and normally require a second subject to be in Mathematics, Physics or Biology. The third A level can be in any subject, although most candidates take a science subject. Most universities will not discriminate if a candidate has chosen an art, language or humanity subject as their third A level as this offers a broader perspective. Occasionally, candidates with two art or humanity A levels might be accepted, providing they have the relevant science subjects at GCSE. It is not compulsory to be studying A-level Biology to gain an offer and there is no disadvantage to starting medical school without it. Such candidates will usually be offered extra lectures and within a couple of months students will be up to speed.

It is very important to check with each institution to find out whether your subject combination is acceptable. Some medical schools will not accept General Studies, Art, Music, Design, Media Studies, Home Economics and Physical Education as a third subject. Also some medical schools do not insist on Chemistry. All this information can be found on the UCAS website.

It is important to have good grades (this means A or A*) at GCSE. Subjects should include Mathematics, Physics, Chemistry, Biology and English Language. If one of the key science subjects (Chemistry, Physics, Biology, Mathematics) is not being taken at A level, candidates must have those subjects at GCSE level. Dual award sciences are acceptable at most medical schools as an alternative to the separate science subjects.

Most medical schools will expect applicants to have a minimum of ABB grades at A level, but some (e.g. Cambridge University) normally ask for three A grades. A few medical schools will accept C grade in some subjects, although this is unusual. In Scotland the equivalent qualifications are the Scottish Qualifications Certificate, or Highers, as issued by the Scottish Qualifications Agency. The Scottish medical schools accept a minimum of five Highers at AAABB but the English medical schools will require three Certificate of Sixth-Year Studies (CSYS) subjects.

It is important to check with each university for the required grades or consult the *University and College Entrance: Official Guide* (published by UCAS). Please note that the requirements may change from year to year and having the required grades does not guarantee a place. You will need to demonstrate other skills and qualities.

As a general rule, the majority of medical schools will not accept BTEC (Business and Technology Education Council) or GNVQ in place of A levels, although some will accept a GNVQ, preferably in science (distinction required), plus an A level in Chemistry. However, the situation may change in the near future. Most medical schools will accept the International Baccalaureate, European Baccalaureate and Irish Leaving Certificate. Some medical schools also accept Access Certificates, HNCs (Higher National Certificates), HNDs (Higher National Diplomas) and qualifications awarded by the Open University, but you will need to check with each school. The full International Baccalaureate at higher levels must include Chemistry.

Employment

In this section, you fill in the details of your work history and employers. If you have not had any jobs, you can leave this section blank, but you will still need to mark it as complete in order to continue with your application.

It is likely that your employment to date is limited to a short time within the retail or leisure industries but, if you are a mature student, you can score points in this section by illustrating that you have been in the employ of a respectable company in a position of responsibility. Enter the names and addresses of your most recent employers, and briefly describe your work, any training you received (e.g. a modern apprenticeship), dates, and whether the work was full time (FT) or part time (PT). You should include weekend and holiday jobs. If you find this section too small, for example if you are a mature student and have had several jobs, contact the universities and colleges to which you have applied if you want to give more information.

Personal statement

Now we reach the part of the UCAS application that strikes fear into the heart of the potential applicant, usually unnecessarily. This is your chance to inform the universities and colleges that you have chosen why you are applying, and why they should want you as a student. Admissions officers will want to know why you are interested in your chosen subject. A good personal statement is important – it could help to persuade an admissions officer to offer you a place.

What to include

This is one of the vital parts of the application. If your academic profile is appropriate, and your referee's statement indicates that you are not a serial killer, then it is all down to this!

One of the key elements of this statement is justifying why you have chosen medicine. You should try to elucidate your motivation for medicine, and any ideas and concepts that interest you about your chosen subject. Try to include any particular interests that you have in your current studies, especially those related to the field of medicine. You should be trying to convince those on the medical school selection committee that you know what to expect from the medical degree course and the medical career that ensues. Include any job, work experience, placement or voluntary work that you have done, and say how it has broadened your knowledge and experience of medicine and helped your own personal development. While you should not undertake voluntary work purely to include on your personal statement, it is a very useful way of indicating that you have done some homework. Remember that you may be asked questions at the interview that relate to your experience, so keep it truthful.

The skills that make a good doctor can seem rather nebulous at times, but certainly good time management and interpersonal skills never go amiss. These are the type of skills that you might have brought into play while gaining a non-accredited key (core) skill through activities such as Young Enterprise, Duke of Edinburgh's Award, or the ASDAN Youth Award Scheme.

Knowledge about medical school AND medicine
Training for medicine normally takes 5 or 6 years. The main choice is between (i) a 3-year university medical degree course leading to a BSc or BA (offered by Oxford, Cambridge and St Andrews universities) followed by a 3-year postgraduate clinical course, or (ii) a 2-year preclinical course followed by a 3-year clinical course at the same medical school and leading to the Bachelor of Medicine (BM/MB) and Bachelor of Surgery (BS/BChir/ChB) degrees. Some medical schools include an intercalated degree within the 5-year course (e.g. Nottingham).

The first option takes a mainly theoretical approach and students have minimal contact with patients during the first 3 years. The second option is more vocational and offers contact with patients in the first 2 years.

Not all medical schools follow the structure set out above, and courses will vary in their approach and emphasis. Medical education is undergoing major change at the moment, with less emphasis on factually based lectures and more emphasis on student-centred learning. In each medical school the curriculum will combine varying elements of traditional teaching, for example lectures, seminars, direct experience and student-led (problem-based) learning. It is important to read the prospectus thoroughly to find out what subjects are covered and how they are taught.

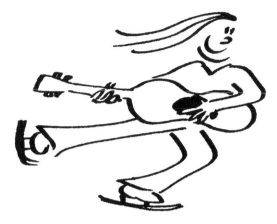

Candidates must demonstrate other interests and abilities

Work experience

Include all your work experience to date. Work experience can be difficult to arrange for students under 18 years old so organizing well in advance is essential; do not underestimate the importance of work experience, especially for graduate-entry students. Work experience is important for showing your commitment to discovering more about a career in the health service. Try to arrange a variety of experiences in both the hospital environment and in the community and with a variety of healthcare professionals. A holiday job as a hospital porter or work shadowing a doctor is always useful, as is voluntary work with children, people with disabilities, the elderly or people with long-term illness. Some people assume that laboratory work would be relevant experience, but most medical schools prefer students to have worked in a more people-orientated environment.

When completing the UCAS application it is important to mention the benefits of work experience, for example:

> I spent a month in the summer of 1995 working as a porter in
> an Accident and Emergency unit in a hospital. This gave me the
> opportunity to experience the kinds of pressures that hospital staff
> are under, to observe treatments, sit in on consultations, and talk
> to doctors and nurses.

If you have non-medically related work experience, talk about what this has taught you. For example, if you work in a shop on Saturdays, mention if you have responsibility for money, or for helping customers or managing people, and how you think these skills will be useful. In addition you should mention any courses that you have attended.

Schoolwork
Avoid mentioning that you enjoy working your fingers to the bone and that you read heavy scientific journals late into the night, every night. Firstly, everyone applying has got good academic results; secondly, unless you are really confident about what you have read, you may be asked a particularly tricky question about it in the interview. Of course, if you have a particular interest in an area of your school studies then this could be a useful addition to your form.

Communication skills
Good communication skills are essential for a future doctor so try to include examples of positions of authority that you have held where your communication skills were important.

Future career plans
It can be worth mentioning any future plans you might have. The majority of those people entering medical school do not have a clue about which branch of medicine they wish to go into, but if you have known for the last 18 years that you want to be a forensic pathologist (a surprisingly popular choice judging from recent applications), then put it on the form. It shows that you have future insight and have considered all the options. However, this could be a dangerous path to tread. How much do you know about the subject? If you know lots and have read widely and considered all the other careers, then it is reasonable to mention your career aspiration. If, however, you just spent a day with a psychiatrist, or just think it sounds interesting, then you may get into difficulties in the interview when they ask 'What particular problems do you think face mentally ill patients in this country at the moment?' Remember it is not necessary to state at this stage which area of medicine you are interested in.

Year out
If you are planning to take a year out, include your reasons why you wish to do this. If you have already made specific plans, include these. The traditional way of spending a year out is to work and travel, but there are many profitable ways of spending a gap year. The subject of gap years is dealt with in Chapter 3.

Social, sport and leisure interests
Most candidates applying for medicine tend to have interests outside academia. This is important when the university is considering your application, because they are looking for students with well-rounded abilities who

have held positions of responsibility. Include all your hobbies and interests but do not lie because it is highly likely that these subjects will be discussed at interview. For example, if you put 'I'm a keen fell walker in the Lake District', be ready to know a few of the names of the fells you have climbed and which of the lakes they are near! Musical and sporting abilities should be mentioned and grades obtained in music examinations listed.

Mature students

If you are a mature student, you should give details of any relevant work experience, paid or unpaid, and information about your current or previous employment. If you want to send more information, perhaps a CV, send it direct to your chosen universities or colleges after you have been sent the acknowledgement letter and application number. Do not send it to UCAS.

International students

If you are an international student, also try to answer these questions. Why do you want to study in the UK? Are you studying any subject that you will not have an exam for? What evidence do you have to show that you can complete a higher education course that is taught in English? Please say if some of your studies have been assessed in English.

Conclusion

End the statement with a few words as to why you feel you are appropriate to be selected.

Points to include in your personal statement

- Evidence of a genuine interest in, and commitment to, a career as a doctor
- Awareness of developments in medical education and healthcare provision
- Demonstration of extensive and varied work experience in different locations
- Evidence of leadership and communication skills
- Evidence of a contribution to school and local community activities
- Demonstration of a variety of non-academic interests and how these activities help personal development

---

The reference

The next section, and one of the most vital parts of your application, is mostly out of your control. Your reference will be added to your application by your school before it is finally submitted to UCAS.

Who should write the reference?

Normally the person writing your reference is the head teacher or similar, but UCAS give guidelines as to whom this person should be. The referee should know you well enough to write about you and to recommend that you are suitable for higher education. Obviously, this person cannot be family, other relatives or friends.

If you are a mature student, this should be a responsible person who knows you, for example an employer, training officer, careers officer, a teacher on a recent relevant further education course, or a senior colleague in employment or voluntary work. Instructions for the person writing the reference are available from UCAS, but normally the person will have written many before.

What will be included in the reference?

Essentially, universities are looking for a responsible person to verify that what is written on the application is bona fide. The referee is asked to include information about academic achievement and potential, including predicted results or performance, whether the candidate is suitable for the course or subject applied for, and any factors that could influence, or could have influenced, performance. They will also comment on qualities such as motivation, powers of analysis, communication skills, independence of thought, career plans, any health or personal circumstances that affect the application, and other interests or activities.

How is this usually done?

Usually the person writing the application will not know you very well personally, but will have a dossier with all the information required to write your reference. All the pieces of information mentioned above will be available from your form teacher, other subject teachers and school attendance. This is then compiled and your reference is complete.

Can I influence the reference?

The usual answer to this question is no, but in reality there are things that you can do to ensure that your reference is as good as it can be. The first is to ensure that the teachers think you have the academic ability to pursue a medical career, and obtain the appropriate grades at A level. Their grade predictions will be based on performance in exams and in the classroom, so a good track record, particularly in mock exams, is vital. The other key thing that you can do is to discuss your career intentions with the person who is writing your reference, which can give you an indication as to whether you are likely to have appropriate grade predictions. While the person writing the reference will not increase your prediction, he or she might be prepared to consider a slightly higher grade if your commitment to a career as a doctor is strong. In short, talk to the people who matter.

2.5 What happens to your application after it is submitted?

Confirmation of receipt

UCAS will acknowledge receipt of your application, after which 'copies' will be sent to each of your chosen universities or colleges. The selection process is discussed in another chapter of this book, but once complete, each university or college will decide whether to make you an offer. UCAS use software to check for plagiarism so avoid cutting and pasting chunks of information from the internet and ensure that your application is both honest and unique to you.

Offers

You will be asked to decide which offers, if any, you want to hold while you wait for your results. The maximum number of offers you can hold is two. Once your results are known, if you meet the conditions of your offer(s), the university or college will confirm your place. It may also confirm your place if you have not met the conditions but your grades are acceptable and there are places still available. If not, you will be eligible for clearing, when you can apply for other courses, including courses at universities and colleges where you have already applied that still have vacancies. Clearing is discussed in the next section. Do not worry about the prospect of clearing – again it is much less daunting than it seems and has a very clear role within the UCAS system. One other point worth mentioning is that UCAS has no say in the selection of students; it is merely an independent intermediary.

2.6 Clearing

Clearing provides an opportunity to apply for any courses which have not been filled; it is available from July to September, although it is most frequently used in August when results are published. You can enter clearing if you have not received any offers or your results do not meet the conditions (usually the necessary grades) of your offers.

   If you find yourself in a position to use clearing, then the list of university courses available through clearing is published on the UCAS clearing website. You can then contact the university and they will consider your application (usually fairly quickly) and then confirm or reject your application. While places to study medicine are not as common as some other courses, places are still available, so it is worth considering this route if you find yourself in a position to use clearing. We would advocate seeking advice before using clearing if possible.

2.7 What are the medical schools looking for?

Having a good academic track record is essential, as medicine is a very demanding subject, but most medical schools want more than just academic skills. Typically, they are looking for the good all-rounder who has wide interests. Anyone who comes across (either on paper or at interview) as an academic swot or as someone who is a bit of a loner may be rejected. Sporting achievements, an interest in the arts and literature, experience of paid or voluntary work, and general life experience are as important as academic achievements.

A survey undertaken by UCAS revealed that most medical schools are, above all, looking for the following:
- an excellent academic track record;
- evidence of a commitment to medicine;
- a well-balanced attitude;
- the ability to think quickly;
- a wide range of interests outside the curriculum;
- competence in communication and interpersonal skills (known as key skills).

In addition, it is important to demonstrate the following:
- a realistic view of the medical profession and what it entails (best demonstrated by work experience, shadowing a doctor in hospital or a GP unit, or through community work experience);
- motivation, stamina and staying power;
- finally, good health.

Remember that medicine is all about communication – it's very much a people profession. Academic high fliers don't necessarily make the best doctors unless they can offer other skills as well.

2.8 How are candidates selected for interview?

The most important selection criteria are, firstly, the predicted grades at A level and, secondly, subjects already passed at AS and GCSE level. After that, the reference and the candidate's own personal statement on the UCAS application are looked at. Anything that makes you stand out will enhance your chances. Not all medical schools interview and for these the selection will be done entirely on the information in your UCAS application.

A candidate needs to show evidence of motivation to study medicine. This could include practical experience of medicine such as spending time shadowing a GP or hospital doctor, or voluntary work. Other achievements to be mentioned should include Duke of Edinburgh's Award, Raleigh International, sporting achievements, school prizes, musical ability or fundraising for a charity. Disclose any interests or hobbies, such as reading, collecting items, making things, being a member of a society, but remember that statements like 'I am an avid reader' are pointless without expanding further.

We have included an example of a personal statement at the end of this chapter. This is not necessarily the ideal statement but is used to stimulate further thought.

2.9 The outcomes and what to do next

Got offer, got grades
Go to medical school!

No offer, achieved 'sufficient' grades
Option 1: apply to medicine through clearing
Option 2: take a year off and reapply

No offer, not got grades
Option 1: consider a non-medical course
Option 2: take a year off and reapply, giving consideration to resitting some exams

Offer, not got grades, etc.
Option 1: talk to the medical school early – there may be a degree of flexibility available
Option 2: otherwise go to 'No offer, not got grades'

EXAMPLE PERSONAL STATEMENT

I have always enjoyed science and, for as long as I can remember, I have had a flair and passion for the subject. I intend to combine this in the future with my strong belief in the need for high class, equally accessible public services. Therefore I wish to study medicine.

I am strongly motivated towards the ideal of public practice and therefore in helping people to improve their quality of life. Empathy, dedication and teamwork are the skills needed to be a doctor. I believe I possess these qualities along with the desire to become a skilled practitioner. Medicine also offers lots of problem-solving, which is something I greatly enjoy.

I am particularly stimulated in studying the Salter's chemistry course, particularly the application of its usage in everyday life. Biology interests me greatly as it explains the mechanics behind the human body and allows you to appreciate how complex we are. Mathematics and physics interest me as much of the course involves problem-solving; physics also offers theories, which make me realize how much we really don't know about the world around us.

I attended a course for potential medics and, through talking to students and lecturers, I gained insight into university life and the way in which medicine is taught.

My commitment to supporting others is evident by the work I conducted with special needs children at a local school. The children were of ages 5 and 6 and had an array of disabilities. During my time there I could visibly see improvements in their communication skills and confidence. This was not only very enjoyable, but also a valuable experience as it made me even more certain that I wanted to enter a caring career. I have arranged work experience in my local hospital during the holidays.

Outside of my academic work I have represented the B team for football, playing as striker. I was part of the sixth form team that staged a charity event which raised £2000 for Cancer Research. I have participated in the school debating society and we recently debated the topic 'Euthanasia should be legalized'. I enjoy playing tennis, badminton and football, which keeps up my fitness and reduces stress. I am a season ticket holder for my local premiership football team.

I am a hard working, honest person who enjoys new challenges. I work in a local newsagent, which shows how I am trusted to handle money and can deal with people. I enjoy this job as it allows me to meet various people. I am approachable with a keen sense of humour.

It has always been my intention to go to university. I believe it is a valuable opportunity where I will meet new friends and develop both intellectually and as a person. I want to use my time at university to learn as much as possible and achieve my goal of becoming a doctor. I am ideally suited to a university environment, with my ability to mix with people from all walks of life, and because I am highly self-motivated and focused on my future.

Universities, courses and codes relevant to medicine

University	Course	Course length (years)	Institution code name	Institution code	Course code	Short form of course title
Aberdeen	Medicine	5	ABRDN	A20	A100	MB/ChB
Birmingham	Medicine	5	BIRM	B32	A100	MBChB/Med
	Medicine (Graduate)	4	BIRM	B32	A101	MBChB/Grad
Brighton & Sussex	Medicine	5	BSMS	B74	A100	BMBS
Bristol	Medicine (Premedical)	6	BRISL	B78	A104	MB/ChB6
	Medicine	5	BRISL	B78	A100	MB/ChB5
	Medicine (Graduate)	4	BRISL	B78	A101	MB/ChB4
Cambridge	Medicine	6	CAM	C05	A100	MB/BChir
	Medicine (Graduate)	4	CAM	C05	A101	MB/Chir4
Cardiff	Medicine (Premedical)	6	CARDF	C15	A104	MBBCh/MedF
	Medicine	5	CARDF	C15	A100	MBBCh/Med
Dundee	Medicine	5	DUND	D65	A100	MB/ChB
	Medicine (Premedical)	6	DUND	D65	A104	MB/ChBP
East Anglia	Medicine	5	EANGL	E14	A100	MMBS/Med
Edinburgh	Medicine	5	EDINB	E56	A100	MBChB/Med5
Glasgow	Medicine	5	GLASG	G28	A100	MB/ChB
Hull/York	Medicine	5	HYMS	H75	A100	BMBS

Imperial College London	Medicine	6	IMP	I50	A100	MBBS/BSc
	Medicine (Graduate)	4	IMP	I50	A101	MBBS/Med
Keele	Medicine (Premedical)	6	KEELE	K12	A104	MBChB/MFY
	Medicine	5	KEELE	K12	A100	MBChB
	Medicine (Graduate)	4	KEELE	K12	A101	MBChB/Grad
King's College London	Medicine	5	KCL	K60	A100	MBBS
	Medicine (Graduate)	4	KCL	K60	A102	MBBS/Med
Leeds	Medicine	5	LEEDS	L23	A100	MBChB
Leicester	Medicine	5	LEICR	L34	A100	MBChB
	Medicine (Graduate)	4	LEICR	L34	A101	MBChB4
Liverpool	Medicine	5	LVRPL	L41	A100	MBChB
	Medicine (Graduate)	4	LVRPL	L41	A101	MBChB/Grad
	Medicine (based at Lancaster)	5	LVRPL	L41	A105	MBChB/M
Manchester	Medicine (Premedical)	6	MANU	M20	A104	MBChB/MedE
	Medicine	5	MANU	M20	A106	MBChB/Med
Newcastle	Medicine	5	NEWC	N21	A100	MBBS
	Medicine (Graduate)	4	NEWC	N21	A101	MBBS/Acc
Nottingham	Medicine	5	NOTTM	N84	A100	BMBS/Med
	Medicine (Graduate)	4	NOTTM	N84	A101	BMBS/Med

(*continued*)

Universities, courses and codes relevant to medicine (*Continued*)

University	Course	Course length (years)	Institution code name	Institution code	Course code	Short form of course title
Oxford	Medicine	6	OXF	O33	A100	BMBCh
	Medicine (Graduate)	4	OXF	O33	A101	BMBCh4
Peninsula	Medicine	5	PMS	P37	A100	BMBS
Queen's Belfast	Medicine	5	QBELF	Q75	A100	MB
Queen Mary London	Medicine	5	QMUL	Q50	A100	MBBS
	Medicine (Graduate)	4	QMUL	Q50	A101	MBBS/Grad
Sheffield	Medicine (Premedical)	6	SHEFD	S18	A104	MBChB
	Medicine	5	SHEFD	S18	A100	MBChB/Med
Southampton	Medicine (Premedical)	6	SOTON	S27	A102	BM6/Med
	Medicine	5	SOTON	S27	A100	BM5/Med
	Medicine (Graduate)	4	SOTON	S27	A101	BM4/Med
St Andrews	Medical Science	3	STA	S36	A100	BSc/Med
St George's London	Medicine	5	SGEO	S49	A100	MBBS5
	Medicine (Graduate)	4	SGEO	S49	A101	MBBS4
University College London	Medicine	6	UCL	U80	A100	MBBS
University of Wales Swansea	Medicine (Graduate)	4	SWAN	S93	A101	MBBCh/Med
Warwick	Medicine (Graduate)	4	WARWK	W20	A101	MBChB/4

General notes

Some of the information contained in this chapter can be altered at short notice. This can include changes such as the addition or removal of courses and alterations in course codes. It is essential to check the UCAS website for the latest information. The usual length of a medical course is 5 years. The courses in the above table marked 'Graduate' are 4-year courses for candidates who already possess (or are currently studying for) a degree. The courses marked 'Premedical' indicate 6-year courses available for students without the requisite science A levels.

Specific notes

Cambridge: The graduate course is only available at Hughes Hall (campus code 7), Lucy Cavendish (campus code L) and Wolfson (campus code W).

Hull/York: This is a joint course. A student will spend the first 2 years at either the University of Hull or the University of York. In the further information part of the choices section of the application form, indicate either for optimum consideration. If you have a strong preference you may indicate Hull or York.

Liverpool: The Lancaster-based 5-year course is campus code L.

Newcastle: It is possible to study the preclinical part of this degree at the University of Durham (Queens Campus, Stockton). The correct campus codes are N for Newcastle and D for Durham.

Nottingham: The graduate course is run at the University of Derby.

Peninsula: Another joint course where the first 2 years are spent at either the University of Exeter or the University of Plymouth.

Queen Mary: The first 2 years are spent at the Mile End Campus with the clinical years spent at Whitechapel. It is necessary to indicate W as the campus code in Section 3(d).

St Andrews: Following the first 3 years of basic medical science, students transfer to Manchester to join the clinical course (it is possible to apply elsewhere for clinical).

Chapter 3 **Admission tests**

3.1 Entrance exams

Entrance exams have been introduced for most of the medical schools. These are evolving and are likely to change in style over the coming years. Two main exams are required: BMAT (BioMedical Admissions Test) and UKCAT (UK Clinical Aptitude Test). Different universities require one or the other exam. This means that you may need to take both exams. The exams are used in shortlisting and in the decision-making process by the universities when considering whether to make you an offer. If you are applying for a graduate-entry course, then things are even more complicated because there are other exams required. Each exam demands an entrance fee, although you may be able to get a bursary if you have financial difficulties.

3.2 BMAT (www.bmat.org.uk)

The BMAT was introduced in the UK in 2003 and has three components.
- Section 1 tests generic skills, including problem-solving, understanding arguments, data analysis and inference abilities. It is assessed by multiple choice and short answer questions over 1 hour.
- Section 2 tests material normally encountered in non-specialist school science and mathematics courses (i.e. up to and including National Curriculum Key Stage 4, double science and higher mathematics). This is also assessed by multiple choice and short answer questions over 30 minutes.
- Section 3 consists of a choice of three short-stimulus essay questions of which one must be answered in 30 minutes.

The Essential Guide to Becoming a Doctor, 3rd edition. © Adrian Blundell,
Richard Harrison and Benjamin Turney. Published 2011 by Blackwell Publishing Ltd.

The exam is 2 hours in length and currently costs £32.10 for UK applicants and £55.90 for international applicants. These fees double for late applications. The exam will usually be taken in your school or college but can be taken in 'open centres' if you are not affiliated to an institution that organizes the test. Full details, including application deadlines, exam dates and practice questions, are available on the website.

3.3 UKCAT (www.ukcat.ac.uk)

The UKCAT was introduced in 2006 and is a computer-based exam. All the questions are in multiple choice format and answered 'on screen'. The exam is divided into four sections.
- Verbal reasoning: assesses ability to think logically about written information and to arrive at a reasoned conclusion.
- Quantitative reasoning: assesses ability to solve numerical problems.
- Abstract reasoning: assesses ability to infer relationships from information by convergent and divergent thinking.
- Decision analysis: assesses ability to deal with various forms of information, to infer relationships, to make informed judgements, and to decide on an appropriate response, in situations of complexity and ambiguity.

Each component lasts between 16 and 30 minutes and will be timed separately. There is an extra 10 minutes to read the exam instructions before the test starts. Therefore the whole exam is completed within 2 hours. Since 2007 the test has included a further component that assesses 'personality' – this attempts to objectively measure qualities such as empathy, integrity and 'mental robustness'. This section, known as 'non-cognitive analysis', is not formally used in the scoring system but provides a simple character report.

The exam currently costs £60 for UK applicants (£75 for late applications). The exam can be taken in any of 150 independent centres in the UK and many centres overseas. Full details, including application deadlines, exam dates, practice questions and the location of the exam centres, are available on the website.

3.4 Graduate-entry courses (4-year courses)

Some graduate-entry courses use the UKCAT and BMAT exams but others use GAMSAT.

3.5 GAMSAT (www.gamsatuk.org)

The Graduate Medical School Admissions Test (GAMSAT) was introduced in 1999 at St George's Medical School for their graduate-entry course. It has now been adopted by other graduate-entry medical courses (see table). The test is in three sections and takes place over the course of a day.

- Section 1: Reasoning in Humanities and Social Sciences. This evaluates ability to think critically, comprehend and reason and is assessed with 75 questions over 1 hour 40 minutes.
- Section 2: Written Communication. This component asks candidates to select two quotations from several on the same theme. Two 30-minutes essays are used to assess your ability to constructively draw together concepts and express ideas fluently.
- Section 3: Reasoning in Biological and Physical Sciences. The questions measure problem-solving aptitudes with regard to scientific scenarios using 110 multiple choice questions over 2 hours and 50 minutes (biology 40%, chemistry 40% and physics 20%).

GAMSAT scores are valid for 2 years, but it is not possible to mix and match scores from different years. Tests are held in September. You must register several months in advance (see website for details). The cost of the exam is £192.

3.6 Summary

Admissions tests are required for entry into most medical schools (see table). Check both the UCAS and individual university websites for details as some universities require more than one of the tests to be taken. Do not underestimate the amount of preparation required to sit these exams. BMAT and GAMSAT require a specific knowledge base; UKCAT may not be testing actual knowledge but it is essential to have prepared thoroughly to be familiar with the types of questions.

Entrance exams required by different universities

University	BMAT	UKCAT	GAMSAT	None
Aberdeen	×	× (A100)		
Birmingham				×
Brighton & Sussex		× (A100)		
Bristol				×
Cambridge	× (A100, A101)			
Cardiff		× (A100, A104)		
Dundee		× (A100, A104)		

East Anglia		× (A100)	
Edinburgh		× (A100)	
Glasgow		× (A100)	
Hull/York		× (A100)	
Imperial College London	× (A100)	× (A101)	
Keele		× (A100, A104)	× (A101)
King's College London		× (A100, A102)	
Leeds		× (A100)	
Leicester		× (A100, A101)	
Liverpool			×
Manchester		× (A104, A106)	
Newcastle		× (A100, A101)	
Nottingham		× (A101)	× (A101)
Oxford	× (A100)	× (A101)	
Peninsula		× (A100)	× (A100*)
Queen Mary London		× (A100, A101)	
Queen's Belfast		× (A100)	
Sheffield		× (A100, A104)	
Southampton		× (A100, A101, A102)	
St Andrews		× (A100)	
St George's London		× (A100)	× (A101)
University College London	× (A100)		
University of Wales at Swansea			× (A101)
Warwick		× (A101)	

* Non-school-leavers applying to Peninsula are required to pass the GAMSAT.

Chapter 4 **The year out**

The aim of this chapter is to describe what a year out (or gap year) is, how it can be organized and to help you decide whether you should consider taking one. Even if you have already decided to take one or not, this chapter still contains some interesting advice. There is a lot of information available about taking a year out, but what needs to be remembered is that potential doctors are facing a 5- or 6-year degree course instead of the usual 3 years, and this has financial and 'age' implications. However, there are enormous potential benefits from a gap year, which can enhance both your university and medical lives.

Traditionally a gap year is taken between school and university. In fact a gap year can be taken at any time and can also be a break from whatever you are currently doing. It can be spent in your home country or abroad; working or volunteering; or merely travelling and seeing the sights.

4.1 The initial decision

Does a gap year affect the chances of a student getting into medical school? This is often one of the first questions people ask. The answer is no, as long as the year is utilized productively. Indeed university admissions officers seem to be getting more enthusiastic about the idea of a gap year; many tutors believe that students start university with a better attitude, not only having matured and experienced more of life, but often more focused and clear that they have chosen the right course. The important point is not to waste it. At interview it will be essential to show that you have thought through the pros and cons and made plans that will enable you to further develop skills useful for your future. A gap year spent living off your parents and doing nothing would not be looked at favourably.

The Essential Guide to Becoming a Doctor, 3rd edition. © Adrian Blundell, Richard Harrison and Benjamin Turney. Published 2011 by Blackwell Publishing Ltd.

Motivation

Students will have differing motivations for taking time out before university. The first thing to realize is that some will have considered it when first thinking about medicine, while others may be almost forced to defer if exam results are lower than expected. After the stress of A levels, some applicants decide a break would be useful to recharge the batteries before embarking on 5 years of further study. Others organize challenging exploits in various parts of the globe either on personal adventures or helping others by undertaking voluntary work. As mentioned above, most plans that you carry out in the gap year will lead to increasing maturity. Whether your specific ideas will help with your chosen profession will depend on the individual. In general, students want to broaden their minds, see new places, learn new skills, find themselves, or simply search for fun and adventure. Multiple skills can be developed during a gap year and some of these are shown below.

General skills	Specific skills
Self-reliance	Language skills
Maturity	Music skills
Teamwork	Industrial skills
Managing money	Work experience
Communication skills	Appreciate culture
Integrity	
Resilience	
Adaptability	

Whatever your motivation for considering a year out, feelings of both trepidation and dread are common. For many this will be the first time away from home and the idea of independence and fending for yourself is often more appealing than the reality. It may not just be you who has concerns; often parents can be worried, so be considerate (especially as they will be helping financially over the next few years!). On the plus side, this is often a person's first opportunity to take control of a significant period of time, without the stress of examinations looming or other responsibilities pressing.

For those not taking a year off, there will of course be a 4 or 5 month gap between finishing exams and starting university and although probably not sufficient for a full round-the-world trip, it is certainly a time not to be wasted. Unfortunately, because of financial pressures, many students need to work for at least part of this time.

A cautionary tale

While most people have a fantastic time in their year out, there may be some for whom things do not work out quite as planned. Firstly, if you make the wrong decision, you may end up bored; extensive world travel does not come cheap and it is early days to be building up an overdraft. If your choice is to remain at home and work for the majority of the year, money may well be less of a problem but staying a further year with your parents may drive you to the verge of insanity – a further 15 months having to live by their rules!

   Some people find work only to despise it, while others may find a beautiful beach in an exotic location, only to miss parents, home or their partner. On a more serious note, world travel, especially if you are on your own or in remote locations, can be potentially dangerous. It is essential that you check with the Foreign Office before planning any exotic travels. Forward planning is essential and travel with friends would be highly recommended. It would be well worth reading a decent guidebook before embarking on such a journey. These tend to be written by well-travelled journalists and are full of tips for avoiding trouble and staying healthy. Good travel insurance is a must; ensure that you are fully covered if you are considering certain dangerous pursuits (e.g. bungee jumping). If you go off on a trip on your own, make sure that people know where you have gone and leave contact numbers wherever possible. To make you aware rather than put you off, some travellers do run into trouble. It is normally through lack of sense. Take the precautions recommended and keep your wits about you, remembering that drugs and alcohol can impair your judgement. The most common problems tend to concern health and often these cannot be prevented – the dreaded Delhi belly! It is worth visiting your doctor before leaving the country and check to see which immunizations will be required. Infections that are not common in this country have an increased incidence in other parts of the world, so don't forget the condoms.

4.2 The options

Whether you have firm plans or just the seedling of an idea, you need to decide if they are realistic. Run through what you want to do, where you want to go and whether your funds match up. Following on from this, decide on how long you want for each activity, but remember to think about your plans for when you return to this country if you are planning to travel.

Bear in mind the feelings of parents and loved ones, and discuss ideas with them. Of course they do not necessarily need to give their permission as you are now 18, but it is better not to upset them too much at this stage.

The main choices for your year off are:
- paid work or voluntary work, at home or abroad;
- travel and adventure;
- a mixture of both.

Gap year ideas

Adventure

Archaeology

Au pair

Chalet person

Charity work

Child care

Conservation projects

Diving trip

Healthcare work

Journalism

Learn new language

Marine conservation

Media

Research

Round-the-world trip

Sailing trip

Summer camps

Teaching English abroad

Tourism

Working with the disabled

Then decide whether you will go with an organized group or completely independently. If travelling with companions, work out an itinerary before leaving to save arguments later. If you are unsure how you will manage away from home, plan an earlier trip immediately after A levels to experiment.

4.3 Practical information about a year out

General

A year out can actually last for longer than a year, usually up to 15 months. For many, it is a time that will not be repeated. You could, for the first time, earn a living, travel the world or make a difference to other peoples' lives. Research into your year-off choice is very important. If you are going to work for the year, then start looking in advance and scout the local papers for appropriate jobs. If travelling, remember that the organization can take longer than you might think. If you are applying for jobs, you may have to produce a curriculum vitae, which is similar to your personal statement on the UCAS form and summarizes your main achievements to date. Another new concept will be that of the tax man – you may be liable for income tax to be deducted from your wage during your gap year. This could also affect payments in future years, so be sure to keep all your wage slips and other important tax documents in a safe place.

For travelling it will be necessary to sort out plane tickets, visas, immunizations, finance, medicals and travel insurance. As mentioned above it would be worthwhile checking various websites and guide books for advice. Visa applications can take up to a month to come through, so be prepared. The other difficulty is that you may well need several visas if you are visiting different countries in a single trip. A useful tip is to photocopy all relevant travel documents – take copies with you and also leave copies in England with relatives. Remember to take the telephone numbers for cancelling credit cards in case of loss or theft.

Funding

This can be one of the main reasons why people are hesitant about a year out. Without doubt it can be expensive but there are ways and means to help. It is certainly worth considering the start of university when budgeting for your year off. It will also be wise to have some money to take to university with you. Travelling the world in first class will be expensive, but the majority of gappers will spend some of the year working and then the rest spending. A useful option is to undertake voluntary work. Many organizations will pay for the travel and living expenses including accommodation. This is a good way of seeing another part of the world without the expense. Don't forget that you will probably be worked fairly hard! Planning is essential at this stage: for example, if you do plan to go travelling, write down all the costs involved and then work out for how long you would have to work to save up this amount. Even if the job is working in a fast food restaurant, you can save a considerable amount of money.

Other sources of money include fundraising and sponsorship by companies or charities.

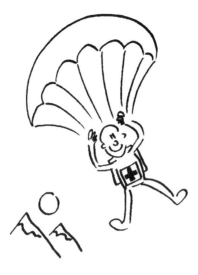

The gap year

4.4 How to apply for a gap year

There are three main ways of applying for a gap year, each having a different strategy attached to them:
- deferred entry (applying before A levels);
- rescheduled entry after A-level results;
- late application, also after A levels.

We would recommend applying for deferred entry. First, contact the university admissions department and find out if they accept applications with deferred entry.

Deferred entry

Simply tick the box (having made the telephone call first) and wait and see. We would also recommend mentioning any specific plans in your personal statement. Also, talk to your teachers to see if they think it is a good idea. You need to convince the university that a year off will make you a better applicant, so give an outline of what you plan to do and why. It might be nearly 2 years before you reach higher education.

Rescheduled entry

If, after A-level results, you have been successful in gaining a place at the medical school of your choice, you can negotiate directly with that university about deferring your entry for another year. Make sure that you check with the course admissions tutor in your first term of sixth form to see if this procedure is OK, before you make a decision not to apply at the normal time. When you have got your A levels, go back to the university and say you would like to take a gap year. If they say yes, you will receive a changed entry date confirmation letter, and you must send the attached form to UCAS within 7 days to accept the place. If they say no, you have the option to take your place or you have to start the application all over again.

It should be noted that this could be considered a risky strategy. Giving up a place on a popular course can be frowned upon, as the university may not be happy about being messed around. Others say that if a course has over-recruited, your deferral will be welcome.

Post A-level application

The third scenario is that you get no offers for the course you want but end up with the grades you need, or that you do not apply in the first place. You may not want to go through clearing for whatever reason, or find no suitable place in clearing. If you have your required grades, then when you reapply (if the university accepts you for your chosen course) you will be made an unconditional offer.

The only other option is that you need to resit your A levels, although this is likely to put you in a position of having to study for the majority of your year off.

4.5 Summary

Whether or not to take a year off is a personal decision, although the matter should be discussed with loved ones, teachers and universities. The traditional reasons for not taking time off revolve around the decision about starting university later and, as medicine is a 5-year degree course, perhaps you should just get on with it. Surely working for 40 years is not much different to working for 39 years in the scheme of things. It would seem that the benefits far outweigh the disadvantages. Of course it is an individual choice and not everyone will enjoy their time. Research and planning is the key as for most things regarding your future. Discuss the matter with students who have done both and get a feel for their various experiences. One thing that is certain is that it will change you, usually for the better. Added maturity, better personal and communication skills, and possibly new practical skills all add up to leading your way to a more successful university life and future career.

Chapters 13 and 22 also have information regarding travel planning and advice.

PERSONAL VIEW *Rick Harrison*

Having been at school for 14 years, the prospect of 12 months of my own time, in which I could do whatever I wished, was quite daunting. At the time, there was relatively little information available on my options, but I had a vague idea that I would like to work and travel.

The number of work options was bewildering, with decisions as to which country to work in, what type of industry and for how much of the year. In the end, despite having a place at medical school, I applied for a job through a company called A Year in Industry, which mainly placed potential engineers with companies for a year prior to university. I had a job interview with ICI, working in a chemical analysis laboratory, and was very surprised to be accepted. I worked alongside existing chemical engineers and laboratory staff on a large ICI chemical production plant, and my job was to check the quality and purity of the chemicals at different stages of production. This involved taking samples from around the plant and analysing them for pH abnormalities, impurities and other criteria. I have to confess that day 1 was very worrying, when I was presented with a laboratory, told I would have 2 weeks' training and then be left to my own devices!

Working for a large company had great benefits, such as access to training facilities; I studied for a computer science course, for example. I also had great fun working with the other analysts in the lab, really experiencing a proper job for the first time. The money was good and allowed me to buy a car and have a good social life. The main downside was that most of my friends who had gone to university were telling me all their stories, which made me quite jealous at the time.

For the last 4 months, I set off travelling with a friend who had also taken a gap year. The trip took a lot of planning, and also a lot of the money that I had saved during the year, but I was determined to see some of the world. We bought a round-the-world ticket, which included flights to Thailand, Malaysia, Indonesia, Australia, New Zealand and America, with lots of overland travel in between. The trip was fantastic and really allowed us to experience different cultures and ways of life. It also provided a sense of freedom, which I never dreamt of while at school or working. The opportunities to scuba dive, go jungle trekking and sail were fantastic and will remain with me for the rest of my life.

Overall, I thoroughly enjoyed my year out and would recommend that everyone take one. Although medicine is a long course, the skills that can be learnt in a year out can be invaluable to potential doctors.

Chapter 5 **Choosing a medical school**

5.1 So many to choose from

In 1997 approximately 12 000 people applied to study medicine at 27 medical schools in the UK and just over 5000 were accepted. Following this there was a small but gradual decline in applications until 2002. Since then there has been a dramatic increase in applicants and although there are more places at medical school, the competition is now greater. The opening of several new medical schools in the last few years has increased the number of institutions offering a medical degree to 31. The table below summarizes the changes in applicant to acceptance ratio in the last few years (source: UCAS 2010).

Year	Number of applicants	Number accepted
2008	18 414	8013
2007	18 597	7837
2006	18 949	8011
2005	19 360	7821
2004	17 826	7955
2003	14 833	7667
2002	11 935	6959
2001	10 231	6240
2000	10 226	5714
1999	10 972	5312
1998	11 807	5119
1997	12 076	5029
1996	12 025	4894

The Essential Guide to Becoming a Doctor, 3rd edition. © Adrian Blundell,
Richard Harrison and Benjamin Turney. Published 2011 by Blackwell Publishing Ltd.

Some medical schools receive over 3000 applications each year. These figures include overseas applicants, who account for around 10% of all undergraduate medical students accepted on courses. Chapter 2 gave advice concerning the medical school application procedure, but the next real question is 'Which universities should I apply to?' There is a vast array of medical schools, each with individual characteristics and idiosyncrasies yet, paradoxically, from an initial inspection of the UCAS handbook, all the universities appear to be too similar to differentiate. This chapter will help guide you through the selection process, demonstrating that, when various criteria are applied, there are significant differences between them; knowing these differences may help with your decision.

5.2 Does it really matter which one I choose?

From a superficial viewpoint it doesn't really matter which medical school you attend because at the end of the course you will graduate with a degree that will allow you to practise as a medical doctor (do not be confused by the fact different establishments offer varying qualifications, i.e. MB, ChB, BM). That aside, there are many reasons to take time over deciding where to apply because the universities can vary considerably – location, type of school, reputation, quality of teaching, format of curriculum, assessments, availability of an intercalated degree and more. While some of these factors may not be important to you, others will.

5.3 How should I go about choosing a medical school?

For applications in 2007, there are five medical schools in London (a few years ago there were many more than this but there have been several mergers and they are now all affiliated to the University of London) and 24 universities outside London that have departments of medicine. Oxford and Cambridge universities also offer degrees in medicine. This makes a total of 31 institutions that offer medical courses. From 2009 there will be 50 undergraduate places available to study medicine at Lancaster University; this course follows the Liverpool curriculum and students graduate with a Liverpool University degree (for those wishing to apply there is a unique course code for the Lancaster course). Applicants to Newcastle University can opt to study at Durham for the first 2 years; interested applicants should apply to Newcastle as normal but place a D in the campus code box.

The UCAS form asks candidates to list five choices of course and establishment. As discussed in Chapter 2, only four of these choices can be medical courses. You should seek advice from your school or college on whether to complete the other slot with an alternative type of course, or leave it blank. Contrary to popular belief, the universities do not know which other establishments you have applied to until the offers have already been made. However, they can see if you have applied to more than one course at that individual university.

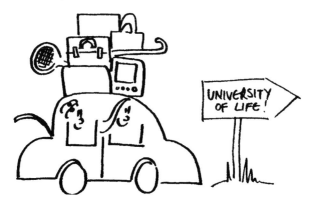

University of life

Medical schools

- University of Aberdeen
- University of Birmingham
- Brighton and Sussex Medical School
- University of Bristol
- University of Cambridge
- Cardiff University
- University of Dundee
- University of East Anglia (Norwich)
- University of Edinburgh
- University of Glasgow
- Hull/York Medical School
- Keele University
- University of Leeds
- University of Leicester
- University of Liverpool
- University of Manchester
- Newcastle University
- University of Nottingham
- Oxford University

- Peninsula College of Medicine and Dentistry
- Queens University Belfast
- University of Sheffield
- University of Southampton
- University of St Andrews
- Swansea University
- University of Warwick

London University Medical Schools
- Imperial College London
- King's College London
- Queen Mary, University of London
- St George's, University of London
- University College London

Things to consider before making a choice on the UCAS form

- Competition for places
- Cost of living in the area
- How easy it is to find accommodation as a student
- Style of teaching on the course
- Assessment methods
- Degree of community-based teaching
- Balance between theory and practice
- Facilities: academic, sporting and social
- Life in and around the university town
- Whether you want to mix with students outside medicine
- Minimum requirements for entry
- Necessity for other entrance assessments

5.4 The factors

Academic reputation

Although mentioned first, it is not the most important factor. While for many subjects, students would be advised to attend the most prestigious university possible, in medicine it is a little different. Whereas Oxbridge is the pinnacle in most subject areas, they offer a different approach to medical education, which will not necessarily suit everybody. Years ago, there was a certain degree of elitism among some medical schools, but the tide seems to have turned with more pioneering medical schools now enjoying a certain degree of elitism themselves, proclaiming that they produce doctors better equipped to deal with medicine in the 21st century. Purely academic candidates do not always make the best doctors. One should consider the medical school's syllabus and teaching methods rather than its reputation.

Traditionally, medical students were placed in a lecture theatre for 2 years and then allowed on the wards for the next 3 years. Most medical schools have designed modern curricula introducing an integrated approach and embracing ward-based teaching much earlier. Places with high academic reputations will be keen to maintain them and are likely to work their students harder, but this does not guarantee that they produce better doctors.

University or medical school?

Universities have the advantage of a large campus, with students studying a variety of other, non-medical, subjects. Most students prefer the mixing of medical and non-medical students during the early years as, during the pure clinical years, it is inevitable that more time will be spent with just medical students. This is mainly due to the combination of other students having a shorter course and medics having little in the way of holiday in the later years. Pure medical schools mean that you will be socializing mainly with medical students, but this could mean a closer knit community.

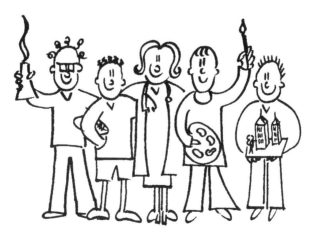

Universities have the advantage of students studying a variety of other, non-medical subjects

Career intentions

Only rarely do medical school applicants know which specialty they wish to pursue. However, there are particular places and hospitals in the country that specialize in a particular aspect of a subject, for example:

- spinal surgery at Stoke Mandeville
- trauma at Birmingham
- eyes at Moorfields
- children at Great Ormond Street.

If you have a true insight into your career intentions, you might consider going to a particular place that will allow you to indulge your career fantasies. We do not think this should influence your decision as the majority of newly qualified doctors will change their career decision following graduation.

Type of course

Aren't they all the same?

Although everybody qualifies as a doctor at the end (providing you have passed!), there are significant differences between the courses. The basic course design is essentially the same, as the medical curriculum is partly dictated by a national body. There have been major changes in course content, methods of teaching and assessment processes over the last 10 years. These have in part been led by the General Medical Council's recommendations for the future training of medical students.

Integrated versus traditional

The traditional method of teaching medicine was to have medical school-based lectures and tutorials for the first 2–3 years and then students would don a white coat, buy a stethoscope and be taught on the hospital wards until graduation. Most medical schools now use a more integrated method and combine these two, previously dichotomous, approaches. In theory, this familiarizes students more quickly and allows them to see the clinical relevance of the theory they are learning in the lecture theatre. There are only a minority of medical schools that keep to the more traditional methods and these often have a 3-year preclinical course which includes a higher degree (e.g. Oxbridge and St Andrews). It is advisable to read the prospectus for each medical school carefully, not least because you will need this information to be prepared for interview at your chosen establishment. It is also useful for determining the actual course teaching and assessment methods. Later chapters in this book deal with life at medical school and the medical school curriculum.

Course length

For most undergraduate medical degrees, the course length is 5 years. If the preclinical course is a full 3 years (see above), then this increases to 6 years. This is also the case if a student enrolls on a foundation medicine course. Graduate-entry courses are 4 years and this is due to shorter holidays and slightly compacted curricula. As financial restraints are sometimes a problem, course length could certainly be a factor when deciding upon choice of medical school.

Extra degree

At most universities there is an option of taking a further year to undertake an extra degree. At some medical schools this is an integral part of the course (e.g. Nottingham University as part of a 5-year course; University College London as part of a 6-year course). This involves a period of research or lecture-based course, and will culminate in a degree such as a BSc or MA. This degree can certainly be a useful addition to your curriculum vitae when applying for jobs. It also allows students to take a short break from medicine or indulge a particular research interest. It is sometimes possible to continue the degree into a PhD, which will take a further 2 years. One other advantage is that if at this stage a student does not feel they wish to continue to the clinical years, they can leave university with an alternative degree.

Town or country?

The medical schools are usually located within major towns or cities, but some are more rural in location. This might have a bearing if you wish to pursue or take up a particular sport or activity. The surfing is not great in Birmingham!

Proximity to home

This is a frequently mentioned factor when people are initially making a decision about their choice of medical school. The prospect of leaving parents, a partner or rugby team can certainly be too much for some, and they choose the nearest medical school. While this should not be considered a mistake, one of the benefits of leaving for university is to gain independence. Living in the same town as your parents and friends can stifle this ability. If you really do not wish to leave your parents too far behind, choose a university that is only a short journey away.

There are a huge number of reasons why a student might want or need to stay near their family. If your only motivation is that you might miss them and it would be convenient to pop home once in a while, we might suggest that you should go a little further afield. Regular trips home to allow your mother to iron your T-shirts may impair your integration into medical school and university life. In some circumstances it may be necessary from a financial perspective to stay near home or even live with loved ones. Again we would advise thinking carefully before committing.

Cost of travel

While we might advocate not living in the same city as your parents, you will probably want to return home during term time. The further away from home, the greater the cost of travel. If travelling from Scotland to Plymouth, these costs could be significant.

Future career location

This is a relatively commonly cited reason for choosing a medical school in a particular part of the country. While some doctors stay in the place they studied, this is infrequent and most doctors move around the country before deciding where to practise long term. Frequently, with the best jobs being very competitive, moving is forced rather than optional. Location can become increasingly important as you climb the career ladder.

Accommodation

The quality and level of provision of accommodation by medical schools varies significantly, although most universities do guarantee first-year students some accommodation. Some cities have plentiful cheap accommodation close to the university but rent can vary considerably and, as medicine is a 5-year course, the cumulative cost can be significant. The relative lack of accommodation available in and around London means extra expense, considerable commuting times and less value for money. While this is not a good enough reason to justify going to one university over another, it is certainly worth bearing in mind. More of this subject is covered in Chapter 9.

Gap year

This subject is covered in Chapter 4, but it is worth bearing in mind that some medical schools can look more favourably on a gap year than others. If you take a gap year, you may want to be with other people who have also taken a gap year. The key is to have organized useful activities for your time out that will strengthen your application to medical school by developing your skills and attitudes.

Strategic applications

Your decision on which medical school to attend should be a personal one. After all you are going to spend up to 6 years of your life there. It is worth noting, however, that some medical schools are more popular than others, and if you apply only to these, you might reduce your chance of a successful application (e.g. the application to acceptance ratio for Cambridge in 2008 was 5.3:1 compared with the national average of 2.3:1). Most doctors we know confess to having made a spread bet application, applying to some popular and some less popular schools. It may also be worth applying to institutions that offer different minimum entry requirements or universities that do not require additional admission exams.

What about my other interests?

Inevitably, you will want to know which medical schools cater for your particular extracurricular activities. It is likely that most universities will be able to cater for you, but check this before you go. While medical school is fairly demanding, there is some opportunity for other hobbies and, with good time management, you can keep several activities going.

5.5 Other options: private medical schools

For students who may be struggling to gain a place at medical school in the UK or who realize their A-level results may not be sufficient for entry into one of the universities mentioned above, there are now some other options. There are a growing number of so-called private medical schools that accept applications from British school-leavers. Despite many of these courses being located in foreign countries, the curriculum is taught in English. Some examples include St Charles University in Prague, St Matthews University in the Cayman Islands and St Georges in the Caribbean. There are also some institutions (e.g. School of Health and Neural Sciences, Nottingham) that run courses in the UK using foreign curricula (usually US). If the course is a US-based 4-year degree, then it would be necessary to complete a premedical year at one of the courses in the UK. The main disadvantages of these courses are the cost and the fact that it is often necessary to sit further exams if a trainee wishes to return to the UK to work (a graduate would be classed as an overseas trainee). The main advantage is that these courses often accept lower entry requirements (e.g. BBC). We would recommend researching these options very carefully before applying. One website worth looking at is www.readmedicine.co.uk.

5.6 Summary

You are likely to have a shortlist of possible universities before you have even finalized your degree choice. Check out the medical school websites, including the student pages and also study the prospectus. Once your shortlist is narrowed down, visit the universities and have a look around the surrounding town and countryside. We recommend attending the open days and talking to as many students and teachers as possible. A common theme when you visit is that the students who show you around will try to persuade you that their medical school is the best in the country (if they don't, then it is probably worth avoiding!). When looking around the university, time is probably spent more profitably chatting to current students and looking around the university campus at accommodation and bars etc. Having a guided tour of a medical school is less useful because the facilities will be similar between institutions (see Chapter 9). It is essential that you talk to as many students as possible to get a feel for the real situation including both the academic and social arrangements. The information included in this chapter can certainly help to cut down your choice of medical school, but at the end of the day if you have a gut feeling, go with it. The odds are that you will have a brilliant time at whichever institution you end up attending.

The best way to find your future medical school is to. . .

- GO THERE!
- Attend the open days
- Meet people
- Talk to current/ex-students
- Talk to staff
- Read the prospectus and alternative prospectus
- Look around the town
- Check out the websites mentioned in the appendix

PERSONAL VIEW   *Zudin Puthucheary*

I am a Malaysian citizen but spent the latter part of my school life and university time in the UK. Since graduation in 1997, I have worked for the NHS apart from a 3-year break in Australia. Times have changed for overseas medical students and if you aim to work here post qualification you must clarify the possibilities of working as a doctor in this country *before* entering medical school. Recently, there have been some important changes to work permits for non-UK nationals. Additionally, in many countries more medical schools are being set up, especially in Southeast Asia. Check that the qualifications you hope to gain in this country will be recognized on your return home. Clarify if you will be required to work in a supervised fashion back in your country of residence and if local graduates will have 'better' jobs earmarked for them. This form of protectionism does exist around the world in medicine, regardless of the quality of your training. Aside from your degree, some countries will expect you to sit further exams on your return, to qualify for unrestricted registration with their Medical Council. In short, think carefully about your long-term plan – if your ultimate goal is to work in your home country but you consider the education system 'superior' in the UK, make sure this will not be frowned upon.

Financial planning is desperately important, especially if you are not studying on a scholarship. Your credit rating will be non-existent, and student life can be hard in this situation when it comes to renting accommodation, hiring cars and applying for credit cards. If you know several years in advance that you are planning to study here, open a bank account at that stage, and if you are self-funded, have your parents do so as well. Regular payments into this account are better than a lump sum for your credit rating. It may help to get a letter of 'good credit' or a reference from your local bank.

A lasting comment from a friend of mine from Malaysia, who also happened to be one of my seniors, was 'Are you going to dress like a foreigner or like a Brit?' His feeling was that there is always a large ex-pat community at medical school, but to really get the best out of my time, he thought I should learn to integrate. The culture shock is often overwhelming and it is natural to turn to your fellow countrymen due to often common interests. However, to overcome this properly takes time and interaction with the locals. I'm told that anthropologists feel at least a year is necessary to understand a different culture! Over the years, while keeping in contact with the Malaysian and Singaporean Society, I made good friends with the British members of my year, and enjoyed my time tremendously. Having a strong support network among my friends and colleagues is even more important with my family so far away. Following university I decided to remain in the UK and complete some of my early professional training as the training and exam structure in the UK is internationally recognized.

That racism is rife in the NHS is agreed – there have been several publications on this situation. It wasn't until recently I grasped the ideology behind institutional racism. I was in Sydney talking to the Australian registrar I was dating when she told me she really had little time for non-Australians, doctors or patients, especially those who didn't speak good English. It struck me that while at work she couldn't see past the cufflinks, Saville row shirt or the (now) British accent, to my skin colour. The NHS employs 1 million people. People are people, good or bad. Racism is not about colour these days, it is about being different, and my European colleagues working in the UK have similar stories despite the UK being increasingly cosmopolitan. My first experience of racism was in clinic when a patient refused to shake 'the darkie's' hand in the waiting room. I dealt with this case calmly and professionally, and every other patient who walked into my consulting room apologized profusely, hoping I didn't believe they were all like that.

So why train here? In my opinion the medical school training here is world class, and the integrated problem-based teaching programmes now seen worldwide take many of their origins from the UK. On a personal level, living in a different country gives you a new perspective on life, and a chance to see very different attitudes, and to overcome your own preconceived views. My advice is to attempt to integrate as much as possible without forgetting your roots. You are living in a foreign country, and you don't really know what your future holds (I've been here for 14 years, still occasionally wondering about going home, mostly during winter!). Medicine is an institution, and you can make great friends, regardless of race, religion or colour. Your friends are also your coping mechanisms, which you will need at more difficult times.
Medical school entry requirements

Medical school entry requirements

University	GCE entry requirements	A levels	AS levels	GCSEs	Graduate entry?	Pre-medical / access course?
Aberdeen	AAB	AAB in three A levels taken together at first sitting over a maximum of 2 years of study. Chemistry required to grade B minimum. One subject from Biology/Human Biology, Maths and Physics required. One further A level in most other subjects. General Studies not acceptable	AS-level attainments do not form part of the academic requirements, as it is on A-level achievement that any offer is made	Grade C passes in English and Maths required. Biology recommended. Physics recommended (or Dual Award Science). Generally, a combination of grade A and B passes at GCSE expected, especially in science subjects	Available	
Birmingham	AAA	Chemistry required plus one from Biology, Physics or Mathematics. One other subject, which could include those named above, but cannot be General Studies or Critical Thinking	Biology required (grade A) if not offered at A2 level	Candidates with AAA predicted or achieved A levels must normally have at least 7A* grades at GCSE, with A grades in GCSE Maths and English	Available	
Brighton and Sussex	340 tariff points	Three A levels. Either Biology or Chemistry should be passed with an A grade. General Studies is not included	You must have studied both Biology and Chemistry to AS level and at least one of these subjects to A level			

(continued)

University	Offer	A-level requirements	AS-level	GCSE requirements		
Bristol	AAB	A in Chemistry and one other laboratory-based science subject. These should be certificated at the same sitting, at the first attempt and completed in 2 years. Avoid undue overlap of content. General Studies and Critical Thinking are not approved	No minimum requirements for AS level	Students must achieve at least five subjects at grade A to include Mathematics, English Language and the sciences. Credit is given to grades at A/A* up to a maximum of eight subjects	Available	Available
Cambridge	A*AA	Passes in *three* of the following: Biology, Chemistry, Physics, Mathematics. One of the subjects must be Chemistry and at least one pass must be at A level		Passes at grades A, B or C in Double Award Science and Mathematics *Note*: Two single awards in GCSE Biology and Physics may be substituted for Double Award Science	Available	
Cardiff	AAB	Three A2 levels, which must include two science subjects from Biology, Chemistry, Physics and either Mathematics or Statistics. At least one A2-level science must be either Biology or Chemistry at A grade	If not offered at A2 level, Biology and Chemistry must be offered with a B grade at AS level. One AS level in a fourth subject (not included in A levels)	The best nine GCSEs are assessed which must include the following: English (grade B), Maths (grade B), Sciences (AA or AAB), other subjects to make a total of 9 at a minimum of grade B		Available

Medical school entry requirements (*Continued*)

University	GCE entry requirements	A levels	AS levels	GCSEs	Graduate entry?	Pre-medical / access course?
		For applicants offering two or more Mathematics and/or Statistics subjects at either AS or A2 level, only one will count towards meeting the conditions of an offer				
		General Studies and Critical Thinking are not acceptable at A2 level				
Dundee	AAA	Including Chemistry and another Science		At least GCSE Biology	Available	Available
		SQA Highers at AAABB including Chemistry and another Science plus Standard Grade/Intermediate 2 Biology				
Durham	AAA	Subjects should include Chemistry and/or Biology at A or AS level. If only one of Biology and/or Chemistry is offered at A or AS level, the other should be offered at GCSE grade A (or Dual Award Science grade A). General Studies and Critical Thinking are not accepted		Five subjects to include English, Maths and either Biology, Chemistry or Physics or Dual Award Science plus one other subject, at minimum grade C	Available	

East Anglia	AAB	One *must* be Biology. General Studies or Critical Thinking not accepted	Plus minimum grade B in fourth AS-level subject	Six GCSEs at grade A, to include Science, Mathematics and English	Available
Edinburgh	AAA	Including Chemistry plus grade B at AS level. A levels must include Chemistry and one of Biology, Mathematics or Physics. Only one of Mathematics or Further Mathematics will be considered. Human Biology may replace Biology. General Studies will not be considered	Biology at AS level required as minimum	Grade B in Biology, Chemistry, English, Mathematics. Double Award Combined Sciences or equivalent at grade BB may replace GCSE grades in sciences. Additional Applied Sciences or Applied Science will not be accepted. All examination grades must be obtained at the first attempt of each subject	
Glasgow	AAB	Three A-level examinations at one sitting to include Chemistry and one of Maths, Physics or Biology	If Biology is not studied at A level, it should be taken at AS level or GCSE (minimum grade B required)	GCSE pass in English at a minimum of grade B is required	Available
Hull/York	AAA	Including Biology and Chemistry. General Studies or Critical Thinking not accepted	A fourth subject at AS level grade B	GCSE Maths and English at grade A plus six other GCSEs at grades A–C	Available

(continued)

Medical school entry requirements (*Continued*)

University	GCE entry requirements	A levels	AS levels	GCSEs	Graduate entry?	Pre-medical / access course?
Imperial College London	AAA + grade B at AS	Including chemistry and/or biology and one science or mathematics subject. If either chemistry or biology is offered alone at A level, then the other is required at AS level	One additional subject at AS level	AAABB or above (in any order): Biology (or Human Biology), Chemistry, English Language, Mathematics (or additional mathematics or statistics), Physics. The science double award may substitute all sciences at GCSE	Available	
Keele	AAB	A-level grades required are AAB including Biology or Chemistry plus another science subject (Maths or Further Maths accepted) and a third rigorous subject. Chemistry as a minimum must be offered at AS level grade B	Chemistry as a minimum must be offered at AS level grade B	Four GCSEs at grade A/A* with English Language and Maths at grade B or better. Core science plus additional science, or any single science not taken at AS/A2, must also be passed at a minimum of grade B	Available	Available
King's College London	AAA + B at AS or AA + AAB at AS	Chemistry and Biology, at least one at A level, the other must be at AS level. If A-level Maths is offered, Further Maths is acceptable at AS-level only		At least grade B at English Language and Maths, if not offered at A/AS level	Available	Available

Institution	Offer	A level requirements	AS level requirements	GCSE requirements		
Leeds	AAB	Including Chemistry at grade A. General Studies and Critical Thinking are not acceptable		At least six grade Bs including English and Maths, and either Dual Science or Chemistry and Biology	Available	
Leicester	AAB	Three of the AS subjects, including Chemistry (grade A) to A2 level	Four AS levels including Biology (or Human Biology) and Chemistry	Applicants must have achieved at least a grade C in English Language, Mathematics and Double Science	Available	
Liverpool (and Cumbria and Lancashire Medical and Dental Consortium)	AAB	Biology (A), Chemistry (A) and one other subject at A level (B). General Studies or Critical Thinking not accepted as third A level			Available	
Manchester	AAB	Minimum grade A in Chemistry (all subjects taken at the same sitting)				Available
Newcastle	AAA	Including Chemistry and/or Biology at A or AS level and excluding General Studies and Critical Thinking		If only one of Biology and/or Chemistry is offered at A or AS level, the other should be offered at GCSE grade A (or Dual Award Science grade A)	Available	

(continued)

Medical school entry requirements (*Continued*)

University	GCE entry requirements	A levels	AS levels	GCSEs	Graduate entry?	Pre-medical / access course?
Nottingham	AAA	Subjects need to include Biology and Chemistry and a third subject excluding General Studies and Critical Thinking		At least six grade A passes to include Chemistry, Biology and Physics (or the science double award). Grade A at AS-level Physics can compensate for a B at GCSE level. Minimum of grade B in Maths and English Language	Available	
Oxford	AAA	Chemistry (compulsory), plus Biology and/or Physics and/or Mathematics to full A level. Excluding Critical Thinking and General Studies			Available	
Peninsula	AAA	Two science subjects from Biology, Chemistry or Physics. If Biology or Chemistry is not studied at A level, this must be studied at AS level. General Studies at A/AS level is not accepted	A fourth subject must be studied at AS level	Seven passes at grades A–C, which must include English Language, Mathematics and either GCSE Single and Additional Science or GCSE Biology		

University					
Queens University Belfast	AAA + A at AS level	Including Chemistry plus at least one from Biology or Mathematics or Physics	If not offered at A level, then Biology to at least AS grade B	Physics or Double Award Science + GCSE Mathematics	
Queen Mary London	AAA + B at AS level	At least two science subjects at A levels, one of which is either Chemistry or Biology, as well as a third A level which can be either another science or a non-science subject	Chemistry and Biology at AS level, and one or both of these subjects at A level. If you are planning to drop either Chemistry or Biology before doing A levels, you must attain a B grade in that subject at AS level	At least six subjects at B grades or above including English Language, Maths and Science. It is acceptable to resit GCSE in English Language and Maths to offer a B grade	Available
Sheffield	AAB	Including Chemistry and another science subject and it is expected that these will be taken in one sitting. The third A level can be in any other subject (General Studies is not acceptable)	Four AS subjects, to include Chemistry and another science subject. Grades of A and three Bs in any of these subjects	Grade C or above in English, Mathematics and the sciences (which may be dual awards). You should have at least six A grades in GCSE subjects	Available
Southampton	AAA	Including Chemistry. General Studies is not accepted	Alternatively, AS-level Chemistry and Biology/ Human Biology can be offered at grade A in addition to grades AAA at A level	Seven GCSEs at grades A*, A or B, including Mathematics, English and Double Award Science (or equivalent)	Available

(continued)

Medical school entry requirements (*Continued*)

University	GCE entry requirements	A levels	AS levels	GCSEs	Graduate entry?	Pre-medical / access course?
St Andrews	AAA	Including Chemistry (A grade) and one other of Biology, Mathematics or Physics		If Biology and Mathematics are not offered at Advanced (A2) or AS level, each must normally have been passed at GCSE grade B or better. Dual Award Science is not acceptable in lieu of GCSE Biology. A pass must also be offered in GCSE English at grade B or better		
St George's London	AAA + B at AS	Three A-level subjects and an additional distinct AS-level subject. All candidates must take Chemistry and (Human) Biology to A level (or one to A level and one to AS level)		Candidates require at least 416 points from their top eight subjects at GCSE, i.e. an average of grade A (A*, 58; A, 52; B, 46; C, 40; D, 34; E, 28). This must include Maths, English Language and Dual Award Science or Single Sciences. GCSE English Language must be at least a grade B	Available	Available

University	A-level offer	A-level subjects	GCSE requirements	Graduate-entry course
Swansea				Available
University College London	AAA + pass in AS	Chemistry and Biology must be studied. A candidate can have a free choice of other AS/A-level subjects except General Studies and Critical Thinking	Grade B or above in both English Language and Mathematics. From 2012 UCL will expect all UK applicants to study a modern foreign language at GCSE or equivalent	Available
Warwick				Available

Chapter 6 **Applying to Oxbridge**

This chapter has been added not because Oxford and Cambridge are better than other medical schools but because they have very different courses, application procedures, and rules and regulations. This can make the whole process pretty confusing.

6.1 The basic facts

First of all, you can only apply to *either* Cambridge or Oxford but not both (unless you want to be an Organ Scholar!). Both Oxford and Cambridge universities are composed of about 30 colleges each. Currently each college interviews its own applicants and awards places at that particular college within the university. This means that you will become a member of a particular college at the university (e.g. St John's College, Cambridge). The total number of medical students is split between the colleges. Not all colleges take the same number of students and the number at any one college varies from about 3 to around 26.

6.2 The differences in the course

Cambridge and Oxford both have quite traditional courses. Students undertake 3 years of undergraduate study before they go to the hospital and start the clinical course. The first 2 years have a compulsory syllabus that covers the basic sciences. In year 3 you undertake a compulsory intercalated degree that leads to the Bachelor of Arts (BA) degree. Oxbridge does not award BSc degrees for historical reasons. Bizarrely, also for historical

The Essential Guide to Becoming a Doctor, 3rd edition. © Adrian Blundell,
Richard Harrison and Benjamin Turney. Published 2011 by Blackwell Publishing Ltd.

reasons, this degree becomes automatically converted to an MA (Master of Arts) about 3 years after you finish your BA!

There are some differences specific to Cambridge. There is an examination system called the Tripos. The first-year exams are called part 1a, the second-year exams part 1b, and the third-year exams part 2. Each year is graded using the usual degree classes, i.e. first, upper second, lower second and third. If you get a first in part 1 (average of part 1a and 1b) and part 2 then you get the famous double first. This is extremely uncommon. Otherwise, the third-year grade is the final degree that you get. If you get a lower second (or better) in the Cambridge exams in the first and second years, then you automatically also pass the professional medical exams (second MB) in that subject and can proceed to the next lot of exams.

In Oxford the first- and second-year exams for each subject are graded: distinction (rare), pass or fail. In the third year they are graded according to the traditional degree grades (first, upper second, lower second, third), and this is the degree you end up with from Oxford.

6.3 The colleges

Currently, the individual colleges are responsible for interviewing you and offering a place. There is ongoing discussion about this and it may change so that there is a central admissions process and then allocation to colleges. Not all the colleges accept undergraduate medical students; check which ones take medical students, how many they accept each year, and how many applicants they received in the preceding year.

The college provides accommodation, dining and most other living facilities (e.g. bar, gym, boat club, tennis courts, squash courts, playing fields, music rooms). The college has a mix of students from all different subjects. Each of the colleges has its own societies: sports teams, orchestras, drama groups, discussion groups, religious groups, etc. The colleges within the university compete against each other in most of the sports, most famously in rowing. In addition to this side of college life, the colleges organize small group teaching (tutorials or supervisions) with often only two, three or four students. These are with a specialist tutor linked to that particular college. This small group teaching is individual to the college and in addition to other teaching organized by the university. This style of teaching is unique to Oxbridge.

Choosing a college is difficult. The first thing to do is look at the college prospectuses, either online at:
- www.cam.ac.uk/admissions/undergraduate (Cambridge)
- www.admissions.ox.ac.uk (Oxford)

or obtain a paper copy of the university prospectus by:

- online application at www.cam.ac.uk/admissions/undergraduate/publications/prospectus/ (Cambridge)
- email undergraduate.admissions@admin.ox.ac.uk (Oxford) and give your name and address.

This will give you basic information about each college. Look at the number of students they take per year and how many applicants they had for medicine last year. The best way is to visit those you are interested in and form your own opinions. The average number of applicants per place for entry in 2008 was 6.1 (Cambridge) and 6.4 (Oxford). Each college has its own atmosphere and, if you feel you fit in, then it is more likely that the people interviewing you will feel that as well. Go to the open days (see the prospectus for details) and see what they say, but also visit independently and browse around the colleges. Speak to the students there and find out as much as possible. It looks good in interview if you can show that you have made the effort and found out as much as possible.

Traditionally in Cambridge, Gonville & Caius (pronounced 'keys') and Downing College have large numbers of medical students every year and the old and famous colleges such as King's, Trinity and St John's are always popular. There are currently about 280 students studying medicine at Cambridge each year. Oxford has far fewer medical students in each year (about 150) and there are no really big medical colleges. Most have about four to six students. The very wealthy old colleges in Oxford are Magdalen (pronounced 'maw-de-len'), Christchurch, St John's and New College.

6.4 The universities

There are no medical departments at Oxford or Cambridge. Each of the undergraduate subjects (e.g. anatomy, biochemistry, physiology) has its own department within the university and students from all the colleges will meet for lectures and practical classes organized by these departments. All medical students will therefore get the same lectures and practical classes, but the small group teaching organized by the colleges will be different depending on which college you attend.

Work aside, all the social activities available at college level are also represented at university level. This means that selection for the university teams is from students from all the colleges. Traditionally, medical students have been well represented in university sports including rugby and rowing. If you represent your university at sport you may receive the famous blue: light blue for Cambridge and dark blue for Oxford. The famous annual Oxford–Cambridge boat race on the Thames and the Oxford varsity rugby match attract avid support every year.

6.5 The application process

The first step in the application process is to register for the BMAT (see Chapter 3). The deadline for BMAT registration is the end of September. You will need a BMAT registration number to put on your application forms.

The next step is to complete your UCAS form and the online Supplementary Application Questionnaire (SAQ) for Cambridge (www.cam.ac.uk/admissions/undergraduate/apply/saq.html). If you apply to Oxbridge you must list *either* Oxford or Cambridge as one of your choices on your UCAS form. The UCAS and Cambridge/Oxford application form must be received before the middle of October the year before you want to start your course. Copies of the application forms should be available through your school. You can either choose one college from the list of those accepting undergraduates or you can enter an open application, which means the university will allocate you to a college.

In Oxford, the last women-only college voted in June 2006 to admit men, making all the colleges coeducational. There are numerous graduate/mature student colleges in Oxford that do not accept medical undergraduates. This is made clear in the advice sheet that accompanies the application form.

In Cambridge, Newnham and Murray Edwards (formerly New Hall) are for women only. A few colleges are primarily for postgraduate students (e.g. those doing PhDs) but accept a few mature students (i.e. those over 21) to do undergraduate subjects. These include Wolfson, Hugh's Hall and Lucy Cavendish (women over 21 only). Homerton does not currently accept medical students.

After you have submitted your UCAS (and online SAQ) form, the next step in the application process is the BMAT. This is taken at the beginning of November, normally in your school/college. The results will be available to the universities at the end of November. In 2008, 43% of the applicants attended for interview. Interviews take place in December.

Timetable for Oxbridge applications

Mid September: closing date for requests for special versions of BMAT question papers (Braille or enlarged text)

End September: standard closing date for BMAT

Mid October: late entry for BMAT closing date (subject to penalty fees)

Mid October: closing date for UCAS applications

End October: online SAQ form for Cambridge applicants

Beginning November: BMAT date

Early to mid December: interviews

End December to early January: results

NB Check the websites for the exact dates, which alter slightly from year to year

6.6 The selection procedure

To get a place at Oxbridge, it is almost assumed you will get at least three A grades at A level (or equivalent). The entrance process is constantly evolving and further changes are anticipated in the next few years. At present all applicants must take the BMAT. It is the responsibility of candidates to ensure they are registered for BMAT (see www.bmat.org.uk for information on how to register). You must register to take the BMAT if you want to apply to Cambridge, Oxford, University College London or Imperial College London. Applications from candidates who have not registered to take the BMAT will not be considered.

Shortlisting for interview will be based on previous academic (GCSE) performance, BMAT score and other information provided in your UCAS application. In Oxford about 40% of applicants will be invited to interview at two different colleges. One of the colleges will be the college of first choice (or assignment if an open application has been made); the second college will be randomly assigned. You will be required to spend a night or two in Oxford in mid December in order to attend the interviews. In Cambridge you will be interviewed in early to mid December by your first-choice college (or assigned college if an open application has been made) if your application is successful. No places will be awarded without interview.

6.7 Interviews

First read the interview chapter (Chapter 7) for general advice in this area. The Oxbridge interviews are held in December and have a reputation for being crazy and difficult. You will hear all sorts of stories about being thrown rugby balls and seeing what you do, or being ignored until you say something – these are untrue. Most colleges have two interviews. There tends to be a medical suitability interview with clinically practising doctors and then an academic suitability interview with the college academics. This is designed to see if you are academically strong enough and will fit in with the tutorial style and academic course. In the academic interview you may be asked strange questions to which you don't know the answers. This is intentional. They are trying to see what you can do on the spot under the pressure of an interview and what you can work out for yourself.

Stay calm, be yourself, listen to the question carefully, think before you say anything stupid, and then have a go at the question. You should not be easily led from your opinion if you really think that you are right but should be flexible and not so rigid that you can't accept other ideas. They are looking to see that you can argue a point and contribute to a discussion. Finally, be prepared to say 'I don't know' if you are really stuck! The interviews usually last about 20 minutes.

6.8 Offers

Like all other universities you will be made a conditional offer. This is usually for three grade As in your A levels. You will be notified by post and it usually arrives around Christmas time. Traditionally, Oxford notifies applicants just before Christmas and Cambridge just after.

Occasionally some candidates are considered by other colleges in what is known as the 'pool'. This is a complicated system in which good candidates are offered places at other colleges if the colleges have not managed to find students of adequate standard from their own applicants. This process may delay your offer and may occasionally require another interview.

6.9 Rejection

If you don't get in, try not to despair as you still have two options. Firstly, you can go to one of your other UCAS choices if you are made an offer. You have not failed and will have a fantastic time somewhere else. Secondly, you can take a gap year and reapply the following year. If you applied to Oxford the first time round, you may try Cambridge the next year and vice versa, or you may try applying to a different college at the same university the second time round. Bear in mind that you must achieve a minimum of three grade As at A level to make it worth reapplying.

If you don't get your necessary grades

If you have an offer but then miss your required grades by a small margin it is worth getting in touch with the college and speaking to the medical tutor for that college. Explain your situation and see if they will still consider taking you. It is worth a try but they may still reject you.

6.10 Conclusion

Oxford and Cambridge are internationally renowned institutions and this results in steep competition for places. All the candidates have very good grades at GCSE/AS level and are predicted to do well at A level. The courses are more academic and the teaching is generally more traditional in style. The college system can make things a bit confusing at first and there is the hassle of a different entrance exam. However, Oxford and Cambridge are unique and fantastic places to study medicine. Have a go – it is worth a try!

6.11 Useful information

Cambridge
- General information about the university: www.cam.ac.uk
- Applying for medicine: www.cam.ac.uk/admissions/undergraduate/
- Address for obtaining university prospectus: CAO, Kellet Lodge, Tennis Court Road, Cambridge CB2 1QJ. Telephone 01223 333308.

Oxford
- General information about the university: www.ox.ac.uk
- About the course: www.admissions.ox.ac.uk/courses/medi.shtml
- Address for obtaining university prospectus: Admissions Information Centre, 67 St Giles, Oxford

Chapter 7 **The interview process**

Interviews are the part of the application process that most students dread. The idea of being sat in front of a panel of doctors and/or academics, and being asked to justify why you think you are good enough to be studying medicine at their medical school is daunting. The vast majority of medical schools interview their applicants. Currently, those that do not routinely interview are Belfast, Edinburgh and Southampton.

Things to remember

- You will spend many years at the medical school you attend, so you need to be sure that it is the right place for you. You must choose them as much as them choosing you.
- For UK applicants in 2008 there were 2.2 applicants per medical school place. That's not bad odds!
- Make sure that you prepare as much as possible.

7.1 Preparation

Preparation is the key to success. You need to think about whether you want to go to medical school and which one will suit you, as early as possible. Go and visit the medical schools, formulate your opinions and see if you think you would fit in. Once you are sure that you want to become a doctor, you will need to work on things to put in your personal statement on your UCAS form. This is, in effect, your curriculum vitae (CV) and is your opportunity to sell yourself. The interviewers are not looking for someone who is just academically good; they want students who are well-rounded individuals with a variety of interests. Spend time on your personal statement and get other people (parents/teachers) to read and check it. Occasionally candidates get carried away and in their enthusiasm to impress they exaggerate

The Essential Guide to Becoming a Doctor, 3rd edition. © Adrian Blundell,
Richard Harrison and Benjamin Turney. Published 2011 by Blackwell Publishing Ltd.

and start to make up extra bits. Don't be tempted to do this because if you are found out, your credibility is ruined and you will not get a place.

7.2 While you are waiting

Once your UCAS form is sent off there will be a considerable time (usually months) before you go for interview. Make sure that you keep a copy of your UCAS form so that you can remind yourself about what you wrote before the interview. Use the time between sending off your UCAS form and the interviews to practise what you are going to say. Get your teachers/parents/friends to arrange mock interviews. Take this seriously and listen to the feedback that the interviewers provide. You can improve your interview style and answers with practice. It will feel more natural on the day, and will often mean that you have formulated the answers and heard them out loud before the real thing. You can also practise on your own by asking yourself a simple straightforward question like 'Why do you want to be a doctor?' and then answering out loud. The first time it will seem strange and you will make a real mess of the answer, but after a couple of goes it becomes more natural.

7.3 On the day of the interview

You will receive a request for interview by post from the medical schools. This will outline where and when your interview(s) will take place. Hopefully you will have visited the medical school before so you will know roughly where you are going. Allow plenty of time to get to your interview – travel the night before if necessary. If you miss your appointment time you may not be offered an alternative.

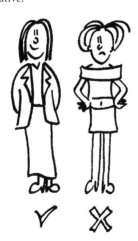

At interview . . . dress to look like a doctor

What to wear

The advice in the letter from the medical school usually says something like 'Wear what you feel comfortable in'. This is standard advice for applicants of all subjects. However, you are applying to be a doctor, and will be interviewed by doctors and consequently are expected to project the image of a doctor. Why make things awkward? It is better to be too smart than underdressed. You will feel more confident if you are smart, and are less likely to feel uncomfortable or embarrassed.

Men could wear a shirt and tie, with smart trousers and a jacket, or a plain suit, with polished shoes. It is more difficult to be specific about women but either smart trousers or a skirt of decent length, and a smart top of some description, or a suit and shirt, will be regarded as suitable. If you don't have such things in your wardrobe then it's worth getting them – it is a small cost in comparison to 5 or 6 years at medical school and you will need them again anyway. You should avoid jeans, way-out clothing, too much in the way of facial and ear piercing, and overpowering aftershaves and perfumes. Imagine what you would like your own doctor to look like when you visit the clinic. This is not to say that you must not wear more casual clothes but why take unnecessary chances?

Before the interview

You will often be waiting around for several hours and sometimes more than one day to be interviewed. There will be lots of other candidates who are all as nervous as you. Try to remain calm. There is usually lots of talk about other interviews, what A levels you are doing/have done, whether you have offers from other universities, and lots of tall stories about the questions that people got asked in previous years/interviews. It is easy to let this worry you but try not to get rattled.

When it is time for your interview, make sure that you are early. If you arrive late, you will be flustered and unable to present yourself in the best way, and it creates a bad impression. Get to the place where the interviews are being held in good time, and wait quietly outside. This will allow you time to prepare yourself.

Preparation on the day of the interview

- Dress and look like a doctor
- Know where you need to be and when
- Be early
- Remain calm
- Don't let others panic you

What do the interviewers know about you before the interview?

The interviewers will usually have received copies of your UCAS form, although this does not happen at all medical schools. On this are your personal details such as name, age and address; your qualifications, and the subjects you are planning to take; your personal statement; and a reference from your head teacher/teachers/sponsor. Often the reference is written by your teachers and then the head teacher will write an introduction and conclusion. Usually teachers write what grade you are predicted to get in each subject. The medical school will take any negative comments seriously. The interviewers will not be aware of your other UCAS choices because these are removed before the form is sent to the university.

7.4 The interview itself

The structure of the interview(s)

Usually you will have one or two interviews and there will be two or three people on the interview panel, although sometimes there may be more. The interviewers will be a mix of academics (who teach basic sciences in the undergraduate curriculum) and clinicians (such as GPs and hospital doctors). In addition there may be a medical student or lay person on the panel. The interviews are usually about 20 to 30 minutes long.

There is some talk of introducing multiple mini-interviews in medical schools. This approach was developed in McMaster University, Canada and comprises up to 10 stations. At each station the candidate is given 2 minutes to read through some material before being interviewed for 8 minutes. This is designed to be objective and to cover common themes mentioned below such as ethics, communication skills and critical thinking. Currently only the University of East Anglia uses this form of interview but it is likely to become more widespread.

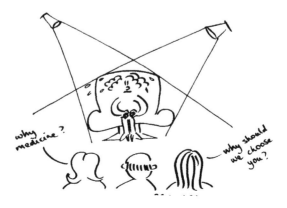

The interview process

Interview etiquette

By this we mean how you should present yourself during the interview. Remember that body language contributes about 70% of communication; in other words, 70% of communication is non-verbal. How you look and behave can be as important as what you say.

On arrival you will be introduced to the panel of interviewers. Shake hands with the panel if you are given the chance, look them in the eye and say 'Good morning' or 'Good afternoon' or 'Hello' as appropriate. Wait to be invited to sit down in the correct chair.

When sitting, adopt an interested posture – sitting upright in the chair, leaning forward slightly and looking ready for the first question. Do not loll in the chair as if you are watching TV at home. Do not cross your legs. Do not fidget or fiddle with things in your pockets or hands, even if you are nervous. These things are all distracting and irritating for the interviewers. Make sure that you speak clearly and at a reasonable pace – don't babble or waffle! Listen carefully to the question and answer the question you are asked, not the one you would rather answer. At the end of the interview you should stand up and shake hands before leaving.

What are they looking for?

Interviewers are looking for students who are academically capable, well motivated and show the appropriate attributes of a doctor. The following tables are examples of attributes that interviewers are trying to assess. This format is used at Oxbridge, where a candidate would have two interviews, but aspects from these tables will be used to assess students at all interviews.

Academic potential interview

Candidate's name:
Criterion
	Score (where a = first rate;
	b = good; c = average;
	d = below average;
	e = very weak)

Reasoning ability: ability to analyse and solve problems using logical and critical approaches	
Originality and creativity of thought: lateral thinking and hypothesis generation	
Speed of thinking and responding	
Spirit of enquiry: keenness to understand the reason for observations; depth; tendency to look for meaning; enthusiasm and curiosity in science	
Observation: accurate, critical, quantitative	

(continued)

Academic potential interview (*Continued*)

Communication: in a tutorial context; willingness and
   ability to express clearly and effectively; ability to
   listen; compatibility with tutorial format
Other factors
Overall assessment (taking above into account
   but not following a strict algorithm)

Medicine suitability interview

Candidate's name: Criterion	Score (where a = acceptable; u = unacceptable)
Empathy: ability and willingness to imagine the feelings of others and understand the reasons for the views of others	
Motivation: a reasonably well informed and strong desire to practise medicine	
Communication: ability to clarify knowledge and ideas using language appropriate to the audience	
Honesty and integrity	
Ethical awareness	
Other factors: ability to work with others; capacity for sustained and intense work	
Overall assessment	

7.5 What are you going to be asked?

This is the big question! Every year the interviewers try to think of new
questions that they can ask the candidates to try to test them. In general
they will start by trying to put you at ease. It is usual for one of the interviewers to run through aspects of your personal statement. This is why it
is important to study a copy before interview and also why it is essential
not to lie or exaggerate. Following this they will move on to more general
questioning, which could be divided into various topics as set out below.
Of course it is impossible to guarantee that these are the questions that you
will be asked, but these suggestions have been included to stimulate further
thought.

Medical questions
About your choice of medicine and medical school
• Why do you want to be a doctor?
• Did anyone you know influence your choice of career?

- Do you have family members who are doctors? What do they think of the field? How have their lives changed over the past few years with the changes in medicine? Do you want to follow in their footsteps?
- Which field of medicine are you interested in?
- Why did you apply to our university?
- Are you aware of the differences in our course compared with other courses? Do you think these should be changed? How would you change them?
- Why should we choose you?
- What are your strengths and weaknesses? What would you change about yourself?
- What qualities would you look for in a doctor?

About the NHS

The NHS has been in existence for over 60 years. It is a British institution that defines healthcare in this country. The NHS is the biggest employer in Europe. Almost all doctors are employed by the NHS for the whole of their career. It is important that you have a working knowledge of what it is, what it stands for and its shortcomings before your interview. Information is available every day in the media.

- What are the principles of the NHS?
- Do you think that the NHS will exist when you qualify?
- If you were in charge, how would you fund healthcare in this country?
- What do you think is the most difficult issue facing the medical community?
- Do you think those who can afford private medical cover should be forced to have it?
- Tell me about a recent media issue involving the NHS.
- Do you know of any changes in the future training of doctors?
- If you can afford it, do you think you should be able to get better care by going privately?
- What would you prefer in a doctor? Bad communication skills with good clinical skills or good communication skills with bad clinical skills? Why?
- Why do you think we hear so much about the NHS and doctors in the media?
- Do you think doctors and the NHS get a bad press, and if so, why?
- What does the current government see as the national priorities in healthcare? Do you agree with these?
- How should the health service achieve a balance between promoting good health and in treating ill health?
- What do you think are the similarities and differences between being a doctor today and being a doctor 50 years ago?
- What does the term 'inequalities in health' mean to you?

- What do you think is the purpose of the health service in the 21st century?
- What do you think are the chief difficulties faced by doctors in their work?
- What do you understand by the term 'holistic medicine'? Do you think it falls within the remit of the NHS?
- Do you think the bulk of medical treatment takes place in hospital or in the community? What makes you think this?
- What do you think is the greatest threat to the health of the British population today?
- Ten years ago most doctors in hospitals wore white coats; now few do. Why do you think this is? What do you think are the arguments for and against white coats?
- Do you think more doctors or more nurses would be of greatest benefit to the nation's health?

Ethical issues

Ethics in healthcare has been summarized in five principles.
- Healthcare is a human right.
- The care of individuals is at the centre of healthcare delivery but must be viewed and practised within the overall context of continuing work to generate the greatest possible health gains for groups and populations.
- The responsibilities of the healthcare delivery system include the prevention of illness and the alleviation of disability.
- Cooperation with each other and those served is imperative for those working within the healthcare delivery system.
- All individuals and groups involved in healthcare, whether providing access or services, have the continuing responsibility to help improve its quality.

Questions concerning ethical issues usually relate to these topics.
- What would you do if you saw a fellow medical student/friend cheating in an exam?
- If an HIV-positive patient was bleeding profusely from a laceration, what would you do? What if you do not have gloves? What if you have an open sore on your hands?
- Should smokers/alcoholics be offered the same rights to treatment? What if they refuse to give up?
- What do you understand by euthanasia? Does euthanasia have a role in modern medicine?
- What do you think of herbal/alternative medicine? Should people choose them over traditional medicine? What would you do if a family member

decided to depend solely on alternative medicine for his treatment of a significant illness (e.g. cancer)?
- Convince me that smoking cannabis should be made legal.
- Is it better to give healthcare or aid to impoverished countries? What do you think about the activities of the charity Medecins sans Frontières?
- Why do you think it is that we cannot give a guarantee that a medical or surgical procedure will be successful?
- What are the differences between length of life and quality of life?
- Should alternative or complementary medicine be funded by the NHS, and why?
- Should the NHS be involved in non-essential surgery/IVF treatment?
- Would you prescribe the oral contraceptive pill to a 14-year-old girl who is sleeping with her boyfriend?
- Is it right that Viagra should only be available to certain groups of men?
- What do you think about the use of animals for testing new drugs?
- A man refuses treatment for a potentially life-threatening condition. What are the ethical issues involved?
- A woman who is bleeding heavily refuses to receive a blood transfusion that you are proposing. Why do you think this might be? How would you handle the issue?
- You have one dialysis machine to share between three patients with equal medical need. One is a 17-year-old drug addict who has just over-dosed, one is a 40-year-old woman with terminal breast cancer and only 6 months of life expectancy, and the third is a 70-year-old marathon runner. Who gets the machine?

Science questions

These are infinite in their scope and are usually designed to see how well you can think on the spot. Some examples are listed below.
- If I release a balloon full of air and allow it to go flying around the room, draw a graph of pressure in the balloon against time?
- What is 12 times 16? How did you calculate this?
- Why do we have seasons?
- Why is it harder to breathe at altitude?
- How do bicycle gears work?
- Do mitochondria have DNA? Why/why not? Could they reproduce in isolation?
- Discuss something that you know a lot about?

The interviewers are not looking to see if you have previously learnt the answers to these questions, they are trying to see if you can work out the answer by logical thought and they will usually guide you through if necessary. They want to see how you approach the questions.

Sometimes props will be used, for example a bone, a surgical instrument or an X-ray. Again you are not expected to know everything but to be able to talk in a sensible and constructive way.

Extracurricular activities
- Do you plan to continue your hobbies through medical school?
- If you had one day to do anything, what would you do?
- What was the last book you read? What did you think about it? Would you recommend that I read it? The last movie you saw? What did you think of it?
- Who do you admire the most in your life? If you could choose one figure in history to have dinner with, who would it be?

Any questions?
Finally, you are likely to be asked whether you have any questions for the interviewers. You do not have to have any questions. It is perfectly acceptable to say 'No thank you, I have been on the open day and spoken with other students and all my questions have been answered' or something similar. It is better not to ask a question that you should have found the answer to at the open day. If you do have a sensible question, you should ask it, but don't ask something pathetic just for the sake of asking a question.

7.6 Differences at Oxford and Cambridge

First of all you can only apply to either Cambridge or Oxford, not both. See Chapter 6 for further details.

Oxford exam

In the past there was an Oxford entrance exam which was sat in schools. This was abolished in the 1990s and for several years candidates sat an exam in Oxford when they attended for interview. This changed again in 2003. All applicants to Oxford (along with several other medical schools) now sit the BMAT (see Chapter 3). Following a successful interview, candidates are now given a conditional offer like everywhere else.

Cambridge

Cambridge did not have an entrance exam for many years and relied on interviews and conditional offers. A few years ago it started to use the

Medical and Veterinary Admissions Test (MVAT) but this was replaced in 2003 by the BMAT (see Chapter 3).

The interviews

Traditionally, the interviews at Oxford and Cambridge have been much more academic than other institutions. Either one or both of the interviews may be dedicated to testing the candidate's academic skills and lateral thinking. The questions are not supposed to see how much you know but instead how much you can work out for yourself (see the Science questions section above). Often the topics are based on things that you should know about, but then try to push you to the next step. Candidates find this worrying and can be easily thrown off their guard. The nature of these questions means that you cannot prepare for them easily. Remember that everyone is in the same position. Try to remain calm, don't panic and think through your answer. The interviewers are trying to assess how you think! Take your time in answering and don't blurt out the first thing that comes into your head.

When you apply to Oxford or Cambridge you may specify to which colleges you wish to apply or make an open application (the university will allocate you to a college). Provided you meet the academic requirements of the college and pass the BMAT, it is likely that you will be interviewed. You will probably have two interviews at any given college. Most colleges now have a 'medical suitability' interview as well as a traditional academic interview at Oxbridge.

Remember that not all colleges have the same number of applicants. The more popular/famous colleges tend to have greater numbers of applicants and this increases the competition. You can find out how many applicants each college received for each subject from the university and college prospectuses.

7.7 The future

Traditionally, selection of medical students has been based almost entirely on academic success. Owing to the number of excellent applicants outweighing the number of places, this has led over the years to the gradual increase in the A-level standards required in order to gain a place at medical school. Even over the last 10 years the average offer has risen from BBB to AAB. This situation may lead to some candidates applying for medicine because of their academic ability rather than their actual motivation for the subject. The admissions tests have been introduced in recent years to try to discriminate between candidates and assess their suitability for medicine.

However, the interview process will probably remain an assessment of academic potential and personality in most universities.

7.8 Finally

Statistically, you have a reasonably good chance of getting into medical school (approximately 2.2 applications per place in 2008). Also there are more opportunities to enter medical school at later dates either as a mature student or as a graduate student on a 4-year course. There are more medical schools and many more medical students now than ever before due to the opening of new medical schools and the increase in the number of medical school places at the other universities. Medicine is a rewarding and fulfilling career, but is also very tough and requires long hours of learning, numerous exams, and hard work. Think carefully, do your homework and apply!

Chapter 8 **Over 21s**

We have entitled this chapter 'Over 21s', as the terminology for the older student applying for medicine can become confusing. The first thing to do is to distinguish between mature students and graduate students. Mature students are those who are older than the usual school leavers (over 21), but who haven't studied for a previous degree. Graduate students are those who have studied for a previous degree and then decide to study medicine. Both groups may be subdivided into those who have done science A levels (or equivalent) or a science degree, and those who have not. There is officially no maximum age for applying to medical school, but as a rule the universities have to take into account how many years after qualifying you will be able to offer as a doctor, and you must be realistic about the cost of training and the potential limits in your career progression if you start at an older age. This chapter should be used in combination with the course code tables at the end of Chapter 2 and the table at the end of Chapter 5 showing entry requirements and additional courses on offer for graduate students and mature students without a science background (Figure 8.1).

8.1 Applications

Applications are through UCAS, using the same form as school-leavers. You can enter four choices of medical school, and it is important that you choose courses for which you are eligible. If you are a graduate you may enter some 4-year and some 5-year course choices. You will also need a reference from your current employer, or if you are a graduate from a recent tutor. You must indicate in your personal statement why you want to apply for medicine, why you didn't apply previously and why you think you would be suited to the course. If you applied as a school-leaver and were not accepted at that time, then you should indicate what has changed since then.

The Essential Guide to Becoming a Doctor, 3rd edition. © Adrian Blundell,
Richard Harrison and Benjamin Turney. Published 2011 by Blackwell Publishing Ltd.

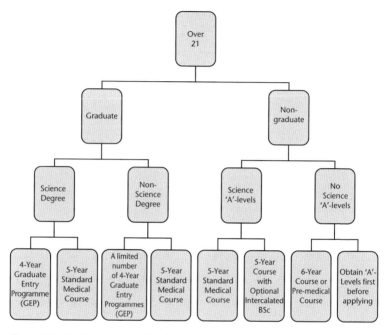

Figure 8.1 Medical degree options for graduate and mature students.

You will need to demonstrate that you have investigated your choice thoroughly. If you are not currently working in a healthcare field, then you must demonstrate that you have been interested and involved in medicine. The most common method is through voluntary work. There are a huge number of organizations that would be grateful for your time and will provide you with experience. Examples include hospice voluntary work, hospital volunteering, St John's ambulance, Samaritans, working as a nurse auxiliary/healthcare assistant, working on social/welfare committees either at university or as community work, working with physically or mentally disabled people, volunteering at a nursing home, shadowing hospital staff or GPs, and working for charities overseas.

8.2 Graduate students

In 2005, 21% of all first-year medical students in England were graduates studying medicine as a second degree. Graduate students who wish to apply for medicine must have achieved at least a 2:1 in their first degree to be seriously considered to study at medical school. Graduates can choose to enter a 'standard' 5 (or 6)-year medical degree but it is now more attractive to try to enter a 4-year graduate-entry programme (GEP). Four-year GEPs have been available since 2000 and have been introduced in many medical schools. Most still require a science degree for entry but many are now including non-science graduates. There are several advantages to a GEP over a standard course. Firstly, and most obviously, the course is shorter and therefore you will start earning sooner. Secondly, the Department of Health will pay the tuition fees for the second, third and fourth years of the 4-year graduate entry course, whereas it will only pay for the fifth (and sixth) years of a standard course for graduate entrants. Also graduates are not eligible for loans for tuition fees and because the tuition fees will be £3290 (2010 cost) per annum this alone is a difference of nearly £10 000 between the two types of course. Thirdly, there are differences in the student loans available for maintenance: GEP entrants can claim a full student loan in the first year and then reduced rates in the subsequent 3 years, whereas graduates on a standard course can claim full loans for maintenance in the first 4 years and reduced rates in the fifth (and sixth) years. Finally, GEP entrants can claim Department of Health bursaries in the years 2–4, whereas graduates on the standard courses can only claim them in the fifth (and sixth) years. There are also grants available to help with travel costs during clinical attachments.

Unlike school-leavers, graduates may apply to both Oxford and Cambridge GEPs. However, the course fees are higher at Oxford and Cambridge. College fees in Cambridge (2009) were around £4500 per annum in addition to the standard university fee (£3290).

Apart from being a shorter course, the courses are more self-directed and problem-based, and have clinical involvement much earlier. It is argued that graduate students are better motivated, but students starting these courses will nonetheless be expected to be very self-motivated and self-disciplined to achieve the same standards in training. These courses are extremely popular.

Four-year Graduate Entry Programmes (UCAS code A101)

Medical school offering Graduate Entry Programme (GEP)	Approximate number of places	Entrance exam	Degree requirement
Barts and The London Queen Mary's School	45	UKCAT	At least 2:1 in a science or health-related degree
Birmingham	40	None at present	At least 2:1 in a life science + good knowledge of chemistry (A-level standard)

(*continued*)

Four-year Graduate Entry Programmes (UCAS code A101) (*Continued*)

Medical school offering Graduate Entry Programme (GEP)	Approximate number of places	Entrance exam	Degree requirement
Bristol	19	None at present	At least 2:1 in a science or health-related degree
Cambridge	20	BMAT	At least 2:1 in any degree + A levels in science subjects
Imperial	50	UKCAT	At least 2:1 in biological degree (2:2 may be considered if offered with PhD or similar)
Keele	10	GAMSAT	At least 2:1 in any degree
Guy's, King's and St Thomas', London	24	UKCAT	At least 2:1 in any degree (or 2:2 if also have higher degree)
Leicester	64	UKCAT	At least 2:1 in a science or health-related degree
Liverpool	32	None at present	At least 2:1 for biomedical/ health science graduates + BBB at A level (including Biology and Chemistry)
Newcastle	25	UKCAT	At least 2:1 in a science or health-related degree
Nottingham	91	GAMSAT	At least 2:2 in any Honours degree
Oxford	30	UKCAT	At least 2:1 in an experimental science degree
Southampton	40	None at present	At least 2:1 in any degree + a pass at A level in Chemistry or passes in Biology/Human Biology and Chemistry at AS level or equivalent
St George's, London	98	GAMSAT	At least 2:2 in any Honours degree
Swansea	70	GAMSAT	At least 2:1 in any degree
Warwick	174	UKCAT	At least 2:1 in a biological science degree

8.3 Mature students

Mature students are generally treated no differently from school-leavers when it comes to getting a place at a university and most universities accept a relatively small number of non-graduate mature students each year.

You must fulfil the same entry requirements as the school-leavers. If you have a science background, then you must achieve the necessary grades for entry into the university you have chosen. If you are from a non-scientific background, you will need to apply for a course with a built-in premedical year or undergo a recognized 1-year premedical training year (foundation courses). There are now many universities offering 6-year courses with a built-in premedical year.

Six-year courses (including premedical year) (UCAS code A104)

Institution	Approximate number of places	Entry requirements	Entry exam
Bristol	10	AAB in non-science subjects at A level, non-science graduates can apply	None
Cardiff	16	AAB in non-science subjects at A/AS level, non-science graduates can apply	UKCAT
Dundee	20	AAA in non-science subjects at A level, non-science graduates can apply	UKCAT
East Anglia	25	BCC minimum in any subjects at A level. Preference given to students from East Anglia and those who do not have personal experience of higher education or a family tradition of entering higher education. Graduates not accepted	UKCAT
Keele	10	AAB in non-science subjects at A level, non-science graduates can apply	UKCAT
King's (KCL)		CCC in selected science subjects at A/AS level. To be eligible to apply you must have been living specifically in inner London and areas of the south-east for at least 1 year. You must also be studying (or have been studying in the last 2 years) at a non-selective state school or college	UKCAT + PQA exam
Liverpool (AZ00)		Normally five GCSE passes at minimum grade B including English and Maths. Apply outside UCAS directly to course (www.liv.ac.uk/study/undergraduate/courses/AZ00.htm)	None
Manchester	20	ABB in non-science subjects at A level, non-science graduates can apply	UKCAT

(*continued*)

Six-year courses (including premedical year) (UCAS code A104) (*Continued*)

Institution	Approximate number of places	Entry requirements	Entry exam
Nottingham	10	CCC in science subjects at A level. The course is for students whose family background or circumstances mean that they are less likely to study health-related courses with competitive entry, or who are from backgrounds underrepresented in such courses	UKCAT
Sheffield	30	AAB in non-science subjects at A/AS level, non-science graduates can apply	UKCAT
Southampton	30	CCC: A-level Chemistry and Biology/Human Biology at grade C or above. Various socioeconomic criteria must be fulfilled	UKCAT
St George's (A103)	20	5 GCSE passes including the sciences (Double Award or individual subjects), Maths and English Language (grade B minimum). Candidates with science A levels or degrees may not apply to this course	None

There are also 1-year stand-alone courses being run, which if completed successfully allow you to apply to medical school (see table below). These courses have limited places for mature students (over 19) and offer variable success rates in medical school admission. Some are only recognized by individual medical schools, some are recognized by many. You have to do well (high marks or distinction) in these courses to be considered and there is no guarantee that you will obtain a place at medical school. For several courses you will also need to complete an entrance exam (BMAT, UKCAT) before entry to medical school. For those that don't make it, these courses provide a foundation to other allied medical professions.

Access to medicine courses

Institution	Places	Requirements	Which medical schools recognize qualification
Bradford	40	GCSE: C in English, Mathematics and individual or double award. A level: 200 points including a minimum of 80 points in a 6-unit science-based award	Leeds: approximately 50% each year transfer to the Leeds medical course

City and Islington College	?	You must be 19 or over at the start of the course. You do not need any formal science qualifications	Five medical schools have accepted students from this course
City College Norwich	Limited	GCSE English, Maths and Science or equivalent The course also requires that you have had 'hands-on' work experience in the healthcare sector	Brighton and Sussex, Bristol, UEA, Hull/York, Keele, King's College London, Leeds, Leicester, Liverpool, Newcastle, Sheffield, Southampton, Cardiff
Lambeth College		Four GCSEs grade A–C or a level 2 vocational qualification, and English and Maths at level 2 in initial college assessment. Some evidence of work shadowing or experience in a relevant subject area is essential	
University of Leeds	5	GCSE: at least six grade Bs including the following: English, Maths, Dual Science or Chemistry and Biology. Preference for local candidates	Leeds
Manchester College of Arts and Technology		Good GCSEs in Maths and English	
Sussex Downs College	11	Good GCSEs in Maths and English	Brighton and Sussex took 8/11 students in recent years
Thames Valley University		A-level grade C in Chemistry and A-level grades C and D in two further subjects, one of which should preferably be Biology. GCSE grade C in English. Certain socioeconomic criteria must be met	Imperial

(continued)

Access to medicine courses (*Continued*)

Institution	Places	Requirements	Which medical schools recognize qualification
College of West Anglia (at King's Lynn)	45+	Five GCSEs or O levels at grades A–C, including English, Maths and Science	Aberdeen, Brighton and Sussex, Cambridge, Cardiff, East Anglia, Edinburgh, Kings, Hull/York, Durham, Leicester, Leeds, Liverpool, Keele, Manchester, Newcastle, Oxford, Royal Free and University College, Sheffield, Southampton, St Andrews

8.4 Summary

The number of graduate-entry medical courses has increased dramatically over the last 10 years. This is an advantage for students who were unsure of their career choice when at school or perhaps for those students who did not score enough points with their A-level results. There is also a variety in the criteria required to apply to each of the schools, with some allowing non-science backgrounds and even a previous degree award of 2:2.

PERSONAL VIEW   *Alex Glover*

In 2003, I was working in London when I was asked what was my ideal job; without hesitation, I replied 'I'd love to be a doctor'. Surprised by my certainty, my friend questioned whether I would consider applying to study medicine. 'Well I did an arts degree and only got a 2:2, both of which narrow my options to get into medical school and I'm 26, am used to having a decent salary and its probably too late if I also want to have a family', I replied. But this conversation did make me think more seriously about my desire to study medicine. With further research I realized it was possible and the need to answer the 'what if' question was becoming more insistent as my career progressed. I finally reasoned that if I applied and gave it my best shot, at least I would have a final decision one way or another.

Having studied every weekend for 4 months to pass the GAMSAT entrance exam (I had no formal science background) and volunteered once a week after work at University College London Hospital, I felt I'd given it my best shot. Thankfully, I was invited to interview and was offered a place on the graduate-entry medical course at Nottingham University. I couldn't believe I'd been successful and was now nervously facing 4 years of full-time study, no regular income and moving away from friends and family to Nottingham!

The first 18 months of the course took place in a purpose-built medical school in Derby, with the curriculum being built around problem-based learning. Each intake varies, from recent university graduates with no employment history to all careers including full-time mums, biochemists and a surf scientist. My background was an Economics MA working in investment banking and then in public affairs. One of the most impressive things about the course was that students had such diverse experience, combined with almost relentless infectious enthusiasm which made it feel that just about anything was possible. In our year group there was an overwhelming sense of collective support for one another, unlike any other studying I have undertaken. Just as well, as it is a steep and intense learning curve especially for non-science graduates like myself, but with everyone's encouragement surmountable nonetheless.

After 18 months we joined the third-year medical undergraduates and started our clinical placements. The first exposure to clinical practice can be exciting and overwhelming and involves a mixture of medicine and surgery. Students are expected to attend formal lectures given by clinicians, clinical skills training, bedside teaching sessions, ward rounds and outpatient clinics. Perhaps as a mature student this transition into the work environment is less intimidating, but any differences among our year quickly disappeared. Regardless of age, to get the most out of each placement you need to be proactive and enthusiastic. The clinical setting is a busy and unfamiliar environment. Having been employed previously, I did find it frustrating to be on the sidelines with no direct responsibility within each clinical team. However, the important thing is to accept the chaos, as this will fade, and to realize that with some initiative medical students can be useful! Clinical placement is not just about putting your previous learning into a clinical context but an opportunity to understand how the NHS works – it's not perfect so it can be frustrating at times! However, you will meet some fantastically inspiring people, patients, families and professionals alike. It is a huge privilege and an exciting opportunity, which I thoroughly recommend.

There are some unique aspects about being a mature junior doctor after graduation, depending on how advanced your age and whether you look your age. Allied professionals, medical staff and patients alike can assume that you have more medical experience than you have in reality, especially if you are

(continued)

(Continued)

naturally confident, so it is extra important to explain your medical experience when introducing yourself in a professional capacity. Equally, there have been moments when I sensed middle-grade colleagues with greater experience may have felt hesitant to correct/instruct/teach mature trainees. I suspect as the NHS becomes more used to mature graduates, this will generally become less novel.

Maturity does perhaps bring greater confidence in dealing with emotional and or complex scenarios on the ward, especially when breaking difficult news. This is obviously subjective and all medical students are taught communication skills for these scenarios, but I think previous life experience can be advantageous when helping patients and their families to cope at difficult times.

Previous career skills that you may already possess, such as presentation skills, analytical skills, committee management, time keeping and maintaining the work/home balance, should be utilized, whereas younger colleagues will develop these skills over time. Equally it is important to recognize that however influential/important you were in your previous career, you are now the least experienced member of the team working in a well-established medical hierarchy. You elected to join it, so accept the step down and enjoy the learning opportunities this presents.

Despite the European Working Time Directive, it is important to appreciate that compliance with the directive of a maximum of 48 hours is based on an average. By definition the job is unpredictable, complications cause theatre lists to over-run, you may have to stay late if patients are very sick – it's all part of gaining valuable experience in the foundation years. This can make childcare or family responsibilities difficult to juggle, so you need to accept that leaving on time is not always possible. Anticipate this by making childcare flexible and not wholly reliant on you leaving work promptly, to make the balance of managing both private and medical responsibilities more realistic and achievable.

Returning to study as a mature student, even if you have a bursary, is a dramatic change of income for the majority. The course is intense and demanding and almost inevitably this overflows into your private life. This is perhaps easier to manage if one is single, but be aware that retraining to become a medic impacts you financially, emotionally and psychologically, and as a result existing dynamics of relationships will be altered. Not all couples manage to adjust successfully, especially if you also throw shift work into the bargain too. The job application process is improving but remains fairly rigid within the institutionalized limitations of the NHS and application timings. As a result, medics can find themselves posted to areas away from their spouse's employment location so be aware it is not as flexible as the corporate world.

Six years on, I am just about to apply for specialist training, and although like any job there are both good and bad days, I have no regrets and frequently see demonstrations of how inspirational the medical profession and the NHS can be. Medicine is a vocation that offers an amazing variety of jobs with unique challenges and rewards so that there is a speciality that will appeal to everyone. I'm also fortunate to know that although the NHS has its faults, the grass is not necessarily greener on the corporate lawn.

Chapter 9 **Life at medical school**

9.1 The beginning

There are those who say that school years are the best years of your life. It is likely that these people have never been to university. University, although hard work, can be a great deal of fun. Whatever course you decide to study, there will be many lasting memories. Choosing medicine gives you a longer course, more students, more societies and more social events. The downside is that there are likely to be more exams than other students, and the longer course can mean increased poverty. A further unique feature is the virtual guarantee of a job following graduation.

For most, commencing university will be the first time away from home. Most universities now reserve a place in a hall of residence (or college) for first-year students. This is perfect for getting to know other students, both medical and non-medical. No matter what your interests are, you will meet people in the first few weeks who will end up being friends for life. Most people will be in the same situation in that they will not know other students before starting. This means that there will be no preconceived opinions regarding your personality before you begin. The advice is just be yourself. The old adage 'children can be so cruel' can be true during school life but once at university the added maturity of students tends to mean teasing and stereotyping are much less common.

What did I think I knew before I went to university?

- University would be good
- Medical school would be extremely hard work
- After 5 years I would qualify and know everything about medicine

---

The Essential Guide to Becoming a Doctor, 3rd edition. © Adrian Blundell,
Richard Harrison and Benjamin Turney. Published 2011 by Blackwell Publishing Ltd.

- Working long hours was only for the first year after graduation
- Exams take place only during university years
- Medicine is a respected profession
- Dissection would be disgusting
- Career choice included GP or surgery
- A junior doctor would always have senior support close at hand

9.2 Accommodation

College rooms

As already mentioned, most first-year students are reserved a place in a hall of residence. For students applying to Oxbridge this will mean accommodation within the chosen college, and for other universities it will usually mean accommodation fairly close to a central campus and medical school. For those students who are not able to gain a place, do not fear, as most will be found places in alternative accommodation that will have liaisons with the other halls. In advance it is difficult to know what personal belongings to bring with you for that very first day. The rooms may be limited in both size and storage area. Most students are dropped off by their parents on the first day with only essential items and then have several trips back home over the next few weeks to pick up the rest of their stuff. This of course means that at the end of the year you have too much stuff for one carload – it is amazing how much hoarding can occur in only one term!

So you've arrived at what is to be home for the next 10 weeks or so. Once the boxes have been transferred to your new room, it is time to gently encourage the parents and loved ones to wander back. Of course there may be tears, but it is time to discover your new environment and meet new friends. Halls and colleges tend to be arranged in blocks with most students having a single room with shared bathroom facilities and a kitchen. The facilities available in the kitchen will depend on whether your particular residence is catered or whether you will be experiencing such literary classics as *Cooking for Students*. The days of single-sex residences are numbered and, as the demand for mixed-sex halls grows, more of the traditional places will no doubt convert. Most halls have central communal areas including a canteen and junior common room (JCR). The JCR is usually the focus for hall life and will have a television and other entertainment such as a pool table and video games. The advantage of living in university accommodation in your first year is that it is good for meeting new friends. It is also reasonably cheap as all bills and quite often food is included. The disadvantages are the size of the accommodation, the lack of privacy and sometimes the quality of the hall canteen.

Renting or buying

Following the first year, the majority of students venture away from the security of halls and colleges. During the second and subsequent years it is quite common to live in student houses with between three and six friends. The quality of this accommodation can vary considerably and so can the cost. It is definitely worth viewing several places before making a choice. Bigger groups of students will find limited availability. Many houses in student areas are substandard despite the introduction of rules and regulations regarding quality and safety. The university will set standards and have a database of houses and landlords who comply. The reality is that demand far outweighs supply. Some towns now have student developments off campus in blocks of flats, often renovated from old warehouses. These are often in good condition and offer a similar social experience to living in halls in the first year. One option would be to move each year and experience different types of accommodation with various friends.

As medicine is a 5-year course, another option in year 2 would be to buy a property. This could be done with a group of friends or on your own with friends renting from you. This has considerable initial set-up costs but could save money in the long run if the value of the house rises. A deposit of at least 10% of the purchase price is usually required and it may be necessary to obtain a loan from your parents or loved ones. The other initial costs include stamp duty, search fees and solicitor fees. As you will not have an income, it will be necessary for a relative to act as a guarantor for your mortgage. The debate about the sort of mortgage to go for (repayment, interest only, ISA, etc.) is ongoing, but advice from several financially astute individuals is recommended.

Once out of university accommodation, the cost of living will undoubtedly increase and this has to be remembered when budgeting. Not only will there be rent but also fuel and phone and food bills.

If you decide to rent then once a suitable house is found it is necessary to complete a contract with the landlord. This should be an assured shorthold tenancy agreement. This means that you will be renting the house as a group and so, if one person moves out, the rest of the tenants could be liable to pay their share. The household bills will need to be changed into your own names and you will have the responsibility for payment. Some students buy individual provisions but an alternative option might be to have communal cooking and hence shared food costs. This can work out cheaper as the necessity for a pint of milk for each individual student will be avoided. It can also avoid the inevitable arguments when someone's last egg mysteriously disappears.

As far as choosing your housemates, it should become obvious during the first term who have become your good mates. Of course there can still be teething problems and some students do swap houses in the following years.

The major gripe will be if one or two friends are not pulling their weight with the household chores. In this instance it may be worth creating rotas for cleaning.

Not all students move away from halls or colleges in the second year, and some actually move back in during their final years. Living in hall is certainly the cheaper of the two options but renting in student houses is another experience not to be missed during your university life.

What did I discover during university?

- University was good fun
- Medical school was not as hard as I imagined
- After 5 years I would qualify and know everything about medicine – how wrong I was, this is just the beginning
- Working long hours exists for most of your career
- There are many, many career choices
- For most careers, postgraduate exams are necessary
- Medicine is a respected profession
- On-call can be lonely, tiring and scary
- It is sensible to avoid hangovers on dissection mornings

Rental survival

There are many horror stories told about naive students being ripped off by dodgy landlords. In general, the majority of students get through their university rental days unscathed. Each university will have a list of approved properties and landlords, and this is a good starting point. This doesn't actually mean that the houses will be luxurious, but means that they must meet certain minimum criteria.

The job of finding a suitable place often requires hours spent tramping the streets, knocking on doors. A slightly quicker method will be to use an agency who can find suitable property for you (they may charge for this service though). Once a house has been found, discuss with the current tenants what the landlord has been like over the preceding year regarding repairs, popping round uninvited, supplying smoke detectors, etc. If they have been satisfied, then arrange to meet with the landlord. All those intending to move into the property should be present. At this meeting discuss deposit, rent, bills and safety checks, and read a copy of the proposed contract. It is probably worth taking the contract away and reading it carefully before signing. If in any doubt regarding the contents, ask a parent or solicitor. Check with the landlord what the deposit covers and that he or she has the correct safety certificates – at minimum there should be a gas safety certificate. Houses should also be fitted with fire doors, mains smoke alarms and fire retardant furniture (check the labels) – again this can be uncommon. On the signing of the contract, it is usual to pay either a deposit or retainer payment. There should be an improvement in the standards of properties since the introduction of the Housing Act (April 2006). If your house has five or more occupants and three or more storeys, the landlord must be registered with the local council and pay for a license. There have also been health and safety systems introduced and if you or your parents are in any doubt about the safety of your accommodation (including university halls), then you can contact the local housing authority if there is no solution to the problem following discussion with the landlord.

When you move into your new home it is essential to check through the inventory that the landlord should have issued. Make sure you agree before signing. If there is any obvious damage, then note it down – a useful tip is to take some digital photos that can be reviewed at the end of the year. All the bills need to be converted into your own name, although in some circumstances (e.g. water services) the landlord may be responsible. Students are exempt from council tax.

At the end of the year, inform the landlord of your date of leaving and clean and tidy the house. Your landlord should then come and inspect the property. Following this you should be refunded a proportion of your deposit. The amount of money lost will depend on the condition of the house. If you feel that the landlord has been unfair, then it is time to study the inventory and dig out the digital photos with the evidence (make sure they are dated at the time and countersigned by a friend if necessary). If the landlord does not return the money, then it may be necessary to write to ask for reasons, then possibly seek legal help. A new scheme to protect deposits was introduced in October 2006; landlords now need to take out special insurance or hand the deposit to a third party. In this way any disputes should be able to be resolved more easily. Any further advice is outside the remit of this chapter and more detailed information can be found at www.nusonline.co.uk.

Rental survival tips

- Check the university recommended properties
- Check the landlord has a license (if applicable)
- Discuss any issues with the current tenants
- Check the contract carefully before signing
- Check safety issues (furniture, alarms, gas checks, etc.)
- Request receipts for all payments made
- Check inventory carefully, take photos, and get witnesses
- Check the landlord is insured *but* get your own personal room insurance

9.3 Freshers' week

The emphasis during the first few weeks at university is not really on working at the books but working on the social life. You will only ever experience one freshers' week, so make the most of it. The week consists of settling in and wandering around getting to know your new university and city. Freshers' fayre takes place during the first few days and is usually found in one of the central campus buildings where the students' union has its home. This involves stalls of all the university clubs and societies that you can wander around at your leisure. There tends to be a diverse number of clubs and examples are shown below. Representatives from companies such as banks, pubs, restaurants and nightclubs also attend these first few days. It is possible to pick up a few freebies at this event but be wary of taking your cheque book on the first day because it involves cash to join most of the societies. It is a great chance to try out a new sport, for example water skiing, but it is unlikely that you will have the time to try out four new sports during your first year. Our advice would be to wander round on the first day and keep your money safely tucked away. Have a look at what is on offer and decide how to spend your money ready for the next visit.

During this first week the university will hold events on most nights. These will usually revolve around the university bars and then some of the pubs and clubs in town. All the events held are usually cheap and cheerful, with the main aim of getting to know new friends. From the social side of things this week often culminates in a university-wide social event, which could have famous live bands headlining and many other types of entertainment.

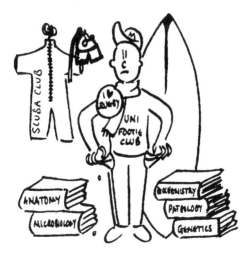

Try and avoid wasting money on too many textbooks or university societies in the first few weeks

Examples of university clubs and societies

- Afro-Caribbean Society
- Anglican Society
- Bike Club
- Bridge Society
- Canoe Society
- Cocktail Society
- Dance Society
- Darts Club
- Folk Dancing
- Food Society
- Golf Society
- Hiking Club
- Lesbian, Gay and Bisexual Society
- Medieval Society
- Movie Society
- Rock Society
- Skiing Society
- Surfing Society
- Swimming Club
- Water Skiing Club
- Windsurfing Society

9.4 The students' union

The National Union of Students (NUS) was set up in 1922. Today the NUS continues to campaign for student rights and offers support to over 700 students' unions across the country. Each university will have its own students' union. These are the backbone of the NUS and are integral to student life. They provide a broad range of services from welfare advice and information to clubs and societies, bars, shops and catering services, and charity fundraising events. Students' unions also play a vital role in facilitating the representation of students' views within the university. Students' union officers often sit on the board of governors of the college or university and help student course representatives at a departmental level as well as supporting students in academic appeals.

Elected student officers conduct the affairs of the students' union and implement policy. Every student has the opportunity to take part in making decisions on policy and areas of work through general meetings or elected councils. In larger students' unions, some elected officers spend a sabbatical year working full time for the students' union, while many unions also employ professional staff. Students' unions decide whether they wish to affiliate to the NUS. Every constituent member of NUS pays an annual subscription fee, which can vary depending on the number of full-time and part-time students who are members of the union and the amount of money the union receives from their college or university. The funds raised from affiliation fees are used to fund the campaigns and activities of the NUS.

The students' union building for each university will normally be found in a central location. The students' union card can be obtained at various allocated places during the first few weeks. You obviously have to provide proof that you are in full-time education. In return for a small fee the card gives you discounts in various shops, pubs, clubs, restaurants and other organizations, for example rail and air travel.

9.5 The medical school facilities

Universities must follow strict guidelines to enable them to set up a medical school. For this reason their actual facilities should not really bother potential applicants too much. Instead of looking round each of the laboratories, time would be more profitably spent chatting to current students, doctors and academics, or even looking around the rest of the university campus and town.

Medical school facilities

- Faculty office: each of the courses at university will be affiliated to a faculty. The faculty office is open during office hours and has many different purposes and personnel. They distribute timetables, organize the exams and generally sort out most problems (or point in the right direction) that students come across
- Histology labs: usually kitted out with microscopes for studying science at a cellular level
- Clinical skills labs: a fairly new initiative for many universities. These facilities allow practical skills to be carried out in a controlled environment, using models (e.g. taking blood from a model arm). Many of the skills that medical students previously acquired by direct patient contact on the ward will now be practised in such environments
- Library
- Computing facilities
- Dissection room
- Physiology labs

(continued)

(*Continued*)

- Biochemistry labs
- Cafeteria
- Bookshop
- Lecture theatres
- Seminar rooms
- Common room

9.6 The first lecture

Of course we shouldn't get too carried away with only socializing in the first week because it is also necessary to begin the medical course. While many of your compatriots may not start lectures in the first week, as a medical student you will not be afforded this luxury. By the first day of lectures you will probably have already met several other medical students and you will now meet up to make your way to the medical school where you will spend most of the next 2 years. The first day will be spent signing on for the course and being shown around the place. Most medical schools have a system in place where you are allocated a 'mum' or 'dad' from the year above. You will normally meet these people on that first day and this may well involve a trip to the local medics' pub. They can advise on all sorts of aspects of medical school. Some will sell you their old textbooks and give you various hints and tips along the way regarding exams and course work. Of course they also know the good pubs, restaurants and where to hang around in your new city.

Before you arrive at university it is possible that you will have been sent a starter pack filled with useful information and suggestions for possible purchases. It is easy to get carried away with buying lots of textbooks either before you begin the course or in the first few weeks. Some people even buy equipment such as ophthalmoscopes. This is not to be encouraged and will be very costly. Most of the books will end up collecting dust on your shelves and become out of date quickly. There is a considerable market for second-hand books which can be a cheap way of obtaining relevant texts, but a word of caution: ask yourself why the second-year student is selling before buying out-of-date and unhelpful texts. Alternatively, the library is a very useful resource and will have multiple copies of the most popular books. Many students buy lots of books in the first year, only to regret their decision. Use the library wisely and also swap books with friends doing different attachments. The advice regarding equipment such as a stethoscope will depend on whether the university you are joining runs a clinical course or a more traditional-based lecture course for the first 2 years. Anything more advanced than a stethoscope will not be necessary. Everything you need you will be able to buy in the first few days once you have arrived at university.

9.7 The medical society

We have already mentioned the various university clubs. As a medical student you are eligible to join the university medical society. This is run by medical students and is exclusively for medical students. The majority of medical students join this society and although membership is not compulsory, it is good value for money. The medical society will have other clubs under its wing, meaning that in your first year it is possible to play sport for your hall of residence/college, medical society or, if you are good enough, the university itself. The medical society also holds regular events that will be subsidized. These will include social events as well as second-hand book sales and elective evenings. Second- or third-year students will normally sit on the committees who are in charge of the clubs and societies that you decide to join. Obviously, many of them need enthusiastic first-year students to get involved with the organization at an early stage and possibly continue with more responsible roles later.

9.8 Charity events

During the autumn it is traditional for most universities to take part in raising money for charity. This period of time is known as rag week and consists of rag raids and further social events for raising money. Rag raids involve visiting nearby cities and collecting money by the sale of rag mags (similar to comics). There is the opportunity to join the charity committees or just do your bit by attending the events.

9.9 The social side

Despite the full working week for medics and the amount of study necessary to pass the exams, most students manage to find spare time to enjoy themselves. How this is filled will depend on the individual. Music and sport are two major pastimes that most students will take part in, to some degree. For the adventurous, this may involve starting a new hobby from the many on offer at the freshers' fayre (see earlier examples). Others may continue their current interests and for some it may even be possible to take these to a higher standard, possibly representing the university or even their country – several athletes in the recent Olympic and Commonwealth Games are current medical students or doctors. Having said this, to pursue an activity to such a high standard will require support and understanding from your university or work place. It is not unknown to be able to extend your studies or arrange flexible training jobs. Some students may find that they do not have enough time to commit to such a high standard and so continue their interests but more as a way of relaxing.

Sport and music aside, there are many other activities to try while at university and more information can be gained at the freshers' fayre. It has to be said that most of the social events will involve alcohol. For most there will be many drunken tales to tell once university has finished, most of them no doubt embarrassing. Do take care as there can be a fine line between harmless fun and people getting hurt. The other point to remember is that although it is reasonably difficult to fail medical school, it is still possible, and it would be a shame for a talented medical student to be asked to leave because he or she didn't know when the partying should have stopped.

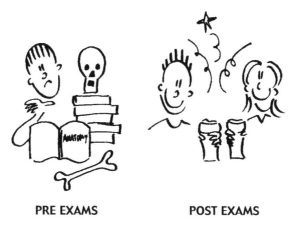

PRE EXAMS   **POST EXAMS**

Life at medical school

9.10 In times of trouble

Of course, for some, the advent of moving away from loved ones does not carry the expected excitement. Some students do find themselves unhappy and this can become even more problematic with a potentially stressful course such as medicine. It is important not to bottle your feelings up. Initially, it will be worthwhile discussing problems with any close friends. If the problems are too personal for this, then a student should approach their nominated course tutor. Not all students get on with their tutor, but most will have found an academic or clinician in whom they can confide. It is possible that the situation may be more serious and, in this case, visiting your GP would be recommended (make sure you register with a new surgery near the university). For those after a confidential ear, most universities provide a telephone service, manned by volunteers. This service often runs in the evenings. Through these channels it is possible to arrange counselling services. Remember that whatever the problem, it is unlikely that it is unique and there will be many people around to discuss the issues – just don't leave it too late.

9.11 Summary

Although often forgotten by more senior doctors, careers advisers and those speaking at courses, university is great fun. The odds are that you will have a good time at whichever university you choose but there is no doubt that medicine can be hard work with lots of exams and assessments. However, medical students do have a bit of a reputation (well deserved) for knowing how to have a good time. Despite the hard work, it is certainly possible to pursue other pastimes and sports. The old saying 'Work hard, play hard' is certainly true. One important piece of advice is that it is essential to have interests outside medicine in order to relax.

PERSONAL VIEW   *Eleanor Dittner*

Work hard, play hard. This phrase, although a cliché, is one I believe rings true for the majority of medical students. My most vivid memories of medical school are a mixture of various fancy dress themed nights with drink-fuelled decadence and panic-filled revision sessions with my close friends before exams.

I arrived at medical school filled with both apprehension and excitement at what lay ahead of me. I was eager to experience what I had aspired to for so many years and yet I was unsure whether I had what it took. I secretly felt that I was the fraud and that everyone was far cleverer than I was. On speaking to my new friends I soon found out I was not alone, we all felt that way, but over the next few weeks and years it became apparent that we were all capable, albeit learning and coping in many different ways. I would say that when I was at medical school I found a happy medium. I was not one to trawl over books endlessly every night but nor was I one of those students who could merely glance at a book the night before an exam and still get straight As. In fact looking back I don't think many people could do that. One thing I can

(continued)

(*Continued*)

safely say is that no matter how much work you do you will always feel you should have done more.

I am sure many people will agree with me when I say that the 5 years at medical school flew by. One minute I was sitting in the lecture being told what to expect from my next 5 years, and the next I was revising for my finals. In between this I had been constantly introduced to new things, whether it was learning how to deliver babies, learning how to take blood or learning how to take a history in Hindi on my elective in India. I soon realized that you never stop learning!

The highlight of medical school for me by far (aside from qualifying!) was the friendships I forged. Medical students have the reputation of being 'cliquey' among other students and I must admit, as hard as we tried, it was often true. The reason for this is that we spent long hours together, whether it be in a lecture theatre, a dissection lab or the hospital itself. We chose to live together in the following years, not only because we were good friends but also because we knew that when it came to more difficult times like exams and deadlines we would understand the need to stay in rather than going out and coming back worse for wear at 4 a.m. in the morning. We inevitably became very close and although we swore we never would, we gained the terrible 'medic' sense of humour. I went through both the most stressful and yet also the happiest times of my life so far with my friends at medical school and this is why, despite living far apart now, we remain so close.

So, all in all, I did work hard and play hard, and now looking back as a junior doctor, it was definitely worth it.

Chapter 10 **The medical course: early years**

The first edition of this book split the following two chapters into the 'pre-clinical' and 'clinical' years. Traditionally, the term 'preclinical' referred to the first couple of years at university. During this time the aim is to teach the fundamental knowledge and principles of medicine, in readiness for the later clinical years spent on the wards. The distinction used to be clear, with little of the preclinical time spent out of the lecture theatre, laboratory and dissection room. These terms tend to be used less now that most medical schools have introduced modern curricula, the main aim being to develop clinical skills at an earlier stage, hence the term 'integrated course'. The aim is to familiarize students with patients, hospital wards and clinical concepts, allowing them to realize the applicability and relevance of what they are learning in the lecture theatre, through hospital visits and patient contact. Unfortunately, this does not mean you have to learn less! The extent of integration varies between medical schools and it is essential to read the prospectus carefully before applying. There are those who believe that early patient contact is irrelevant as the students have too little knowledge, but most educationalists believe this to be a useful exercise, as communicating and dealing with patients and relatives is one of the most essential attributes of a future doctor. Having early patient contact allows essential skills to be learned while the student is under careful supervision.

10.1 Mentor/educational supervisor

On arrival at most medical schools, each student is allocated a mentor. This will usually be an academic teacher from one of the affiliated departments (e.g. biochemistry). Several students may have the same mentor, who should arrange several meetings over the first couple of years. These get-togethers

The Essential Guide to Becoming a Doctor, 3rd edition. © Adrian Blundell,
Richard Harrison and Benjamin Turney. Published 2011 by Blackwell Publishing Ltd.

are to check that you have no particular problems and are progressing with the course, and they often involve feedback following exams. Meetings on a one-to-one basis can be arranged if problems are a little more personal.

10.2 Types of teaching

Regardless of the nature of the course, teaching takes place in the following forms: lectures, practical sessions, dissection, clinical skills sessions and small group tutorials.

Lectures

Formal lectures remain the most common method of teaching. The lectures are usually presented by basic science academics. Computer presentations are the mainstay, with handouts often provided to complement the talks. The format and quality can vary significantly: a university academic does not necessarily have any teaching qualifications. Interactivity can be limited, although the use of audience response keypads can improve this. Lectures are becoming less popular as newer methods of teaching are being adopted but they remain the easiest way of delivering a large amount of information to large numbers of students.

Practical sessions

To help with understanding certain concepts, time will be spent in the laboratory. Here it is possible to apply some of the knowledge gained from the lecture theatre. Practicals undertaken will include experiments in subjects such as physiology, biochemistry, pharmacology and microbiology. Occasionally an academic teacher will run the experiment but more often than not it is time for students to get their hands dirty (hopefully not literally, especially for some microbiology experiments!). The particularly fun sessions will involve clinically relevant experiments that can be performed on each other. One of the less pleasant tasks could be inserting a nasogastric tube (tube passed into the stomach) to aid in the measurement of gastric pH. The practical sessions will often involve a write-up following the experiment, in a similar format to those written during A levels. These may count towards a final assessment.

Clinical skills sessions

Most medical schools have clinical skills laboratories that can be used by students from all years. In these environments it is possible to practise practical skills (e.g. taking blood) and also gain experience of managing acute medical conditions (e.g. cardiopulmonary resuscitation) using mechanical and computerized mannequins and models. Technology is rapidly developing, with mannequins and simulators improving all the time – the latest models have palpable pulses, dilating pupils, audible breath sounds and can even talk to you! These facilities give students the opportunity to improve their skills in a non-threatening environment before carrying them out on real-life patients. The clinical sessions will also involve visits to GP surgeries and hospital wards.

Dissection sessions

Ah, the smell of formaldehyde! It's not all lectures during the first couple of years. A major part of the preclinical curriculum is anatomy. The study of anatomy can vary from school to school so it is worth checking on this before arriving. The options include small group teaching with a donated cadaver which the students dissect, small group teaching using pro-sections (parts of the body previously dissected to show the relevant parts), or teaching using computer-generated images. The best approach will involve a combination. Although we do not recommend purchasing too many textbooks, a good anatomy book will be necessary. The best approach is to read the relevant chapters before the session and so reinforce the information.

The utmost respect should be paid at all times to the cadavers. These people have kindly donated their bodies for the sake of science. There are many tales told to junior medical students regarding the tricks that have been played in the past (placing parts of the bodies in your mate's dinner!). Many are urban myths – if any are true, then it is highly inappropriate behaviour. The medical school authorities will take a strict approach with any student caught fooling around and expulsion would be likely.

Another point to remember is that anatomy is relevant and interesting to everybody, not just the budding surgeon.

Tutorials

The problem with lectures is the sheer size of the audience. The disadvantages are that the talks tend to be less interactive and students can feel more intimidated in a crowd and so not ask as many questions. On arrival at university, students will be split into tutorial groups who will meet with a supervisor up to once a week. At these sessions it will be possible to cover problem areas or present experimental findings. It is also likely that, as students, you will be expected to prepare presentations and hand in assignments. It will depend on the particular medical school as to how much work is involved. The size of tutorials varies greatly between institutions, for example at Oxford there may be only two students in each group. Schools that run problem-based learning courses tend to have more tutorial work.

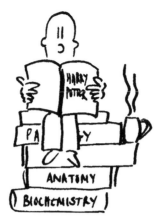

The preclinical years

10.3 Computing

Over the last decade the advances in computer technology have led to increased emphasis being placed on information technology (IT) within the medical school curriculum. Universities will now provide teaching on the use of word processing, presentation, statistics, spreadsheet and data-base packages. Some aspects of the course may be taught using compu-ter-aided learning (CAL) packages to supplement the lecture material. A more recent development is the use of so-called learning environments where the timetables and objectives for the whole of the medical course are found on intranet sites. These sites may also provide lecture material, useful links and sample exam questions. Some centres even run certain assessments on the intranet. Your future career will require increasing use of the internet and IT methods. While at university take the opportuni-ties available to familiarize yourself with presenting talks using presenta-tion packages and perform literature searches using search engines such as Medline.

Universities vary in the degree to which IT is used in the teaching and learning environment. Some universities are embracing patient simulators, podcasting and networked learning environments, which have enormous potential advantages in terms of access but can be costly. If you feel that you lean more effectively through the use of IT, it might be wise to explore the differing approaches and access to IT-based learning. One point worth men-tioning is that medical students will require a degree of computer literacy, but don't worry, universities provide courses to get you up to speed.

10.4 The curriculum

Courses that are more traditional run various subjects each term, for example the first term may consist of a biochemistry module, the second term a physiology module. This trend is changing and the new method is to teach about a whole system, for example in the first term the topic may be the cardiovascular system and the teaching in physiology, anatomy, biochemistry and other topics would be relevant to that system. During this time it is common for several hospital visits to be arranged to attempt to put the theoretical knowledge into place with real-life patients. The idea is to simplify the course and make everything more relevant.

Most medical schools introduce the curriculum over the first 2 years in themes. These themes vary between centres but will include, in some way, basic medical sciences, personal and professional development, patient–doctor relationships, and public health and community medicine. Basic medical science is the understanding of the science behind disease processes. Initially it will be necessary to gain an understanding of the normal functioning of the human body before progressing to the abnormal processes that can occur. This topic is large and will include biochemistry, physiology, pharmacology, anatomy and microbiology. Unlike school days, where much of the teaching emphasizes spoon feeding, at university you will be expected to cover much of the bookwork in your own time, based around the lectures and tutorials that are presented. The other themes introduce, at an early stage in the course, communication skills, evidence-based medicine, population medicine and psychological aspects related to illness. Universities differ greatly in the amount of written work that you are expected to complete and hand in for assessment during term time. Students at more traditional courses may find more assessments of this sort during the term. Other medical schools have few or no essays and practical assignments to be written up, and use examinations as the only formal assessment. Again, it is important, when deciding to which university to apply, that you are aware of the course differences. This can be achieved by reading the appropriate prospectus and talking to students who are already studying at the particular institution. You may have to work harder at some medical schools compared with others!

The early curriculum

- Anatomy
- Biochemistry
- Cytology

(continued)

(*Continued*)

- Embryology
- Epidemiology
- Genetics
- Haematology
- Histology
- Immunology
- Microbiology
- Pathology
- Pharmacology and therapeutics
- Physiology
- Psychology
- Sociology

Anatomy

This is the study of body structure and is one of the very essences of medicine, but unfortunately presents a huge amount of information to learn. It is taught mainly in the lecture theatre and dissection room, but increasingly through small group tutorials and computer-aided teaching packages. This subject also involves histology, which is the microscopic appearance of the different parts of the body, and embryology, which is the study of the development of the human body.

Pathology

Just when you have learnt how everything works and where it is in the body, you have to learn that everything can go wrong, and in many different ways! Pathology is the scientific study of the nature of disease and its causes, processes, development and consequences. It is taught usually through lectures, but also involves attending post-mortems and microscope practical sessions.

Pharmacology

Defined as the study of the changes produced in living animals by chemical substances. Often taught with pharmacy students, this course will teach the mechanisms of action of therapeutic agents within the body and their effects, both positive and negative.

Physiology and biochemistry

This is the biological study of the functions of living organisms and their parts and the study of the chemical substances and vital processes occurring in living organisms, respectively. Essentially it is learning about biological processes and how they occur within the human body. The subjects are taught mainly in the lecture theatre, but study also usually involves small group tutorials and practical sessions. Again there is a large amount of information to learn.

10.5 The early clinical experience

Integrated/systems-based learning

With the advent of some newer courses in the early 1990s it was felt that earlier clinical exposure was probably useful for medical students. Initially this meant that a handful of schools made a token attempt to integrate the course, which often just meant a brief visit to a hospital ward each term. This has become more formalized over the last decade, especially with the opening of the newer medical schools. The majority now run fully integrated courses, although the extent of clinical contact in the first 2 years can vary, so it is worth checking before applying. The experience can vary from a few visits each semester to a local hospital or GP, to a dedicated session each week. As many courses are now taught using a systems-based approach (see above section), hospital visits are often organized for the relevant system at the appropriate time.

As well as hospital visits, students will often be attached to a local GP surgery for the whole of the 2 years. During this time some universities assign students various community projects, for example watching the development of a newborn baby or following the progress of an older person after surgery. This early exposure to patients aims to make the basic medical sciences more relevant to everyday practice. It also assists students to develop their communication skills. As there is now this clinical component to the early years, assessment methods have also changed and students will be required to demonstrate, at an early stage, their competence in various clinical situations (see below). This type of course is run at the majority of UK medical schools.

Traditional/subject-based

Now relatively rare, this is limited to medical schools such as Oxford, Cambridge and St Andrews; there is a definite preclinical/clinical divide and the preclinical years are taught rigidly in subjects. In some of these institutions you may have to apply again for a 'clinical' place and your clinical place may not even be in the city you started, for example St Andrews' students finish their clinical years in Manchester and some Oxbridge students finish their years in London. This type of degree offers much more scope to complete research (such as a Masters or PhD) without overly disrupting your degree. This is probably suited to those who are more 'scientific' and those who like the idea of studying a science degree before embarking on clinical studies.

10.6 Problem-based learning

When applying to medical school you will have considered the merits of each different university and course. Some applicants may be concerned with the range of bars, others with the ratio of boys to girls. As discussed earlier another decision to bear in mind is the type of course, and a concept that you should all be aware of is self-directed problem-based learning (PBL).

At school a common teaching technique is spoon-feeding. Students are told what to learn and given fact after fact. This way the emphasis on reading around the subject is neglected and there is a tendency to cram the knowledge, in order to pass the exams. Medical education has undergone sweeping changes over the last few years and new methods and ideas for teaching are being introduced.

PBL is not a new concept. Its origins date back to France in 1920, with a teacher (Célestin Freinet) returning from the First World War unable to speak to his pupils for very long before being short of breath, due to the injuries he sustained. Owing to this disability he developed methods to get his pupils more involved during the classes. His radical methods, despite the encouraging results, were rejected by all establishments until, in 1969, McMaster University in Ontario, Canada adopted PBL, led by Howard Barrows. The University of Maastricht followed in 1974, and many other centres worldwide have since followed suit. From as far afield as Australia and Bahrain, to right here in the UK, PBL is the new face of how you are likely to be taught at some stage during your medical education. This new method is not being limited to medicine; other subjects to change include law, economics and mathematics.

Basically PBL rests on the principle that crammed information given to you in a didactic fashion, and regurgitated for an exam, is soon forgotten. Alternatively, if a student has to search for the information, it is likely to remain in the memory for a longer period of time. This technique is more suited to the university style of teaching, as information tends no longer to be spoon-fed and the emphasis is more on individual information gathering.

The way PBL works in reality is by having small group seminars. A university tutor will get together with a group of students (usually between six and ten) and discuss some trigger material, which may be a letter, a video or a fictitious scenario. From that, together as a group and guided by the tutor, you discuss issues raised and come up with some learning objectives for the week. You then break up and gather the information for yourselves from various resources such as books, the internet, professionals and each other. When you return after a week, you solve the problems set by sharing all the information you have found, again guided by the tutor. You will often hear this referred to as the adult learning method, and you will learn about the seven or eight step tutorial process.

PBL is a very different style of learning to what you may be used to, but research and experience have shown that qualifying doctors from this type of course are just as capable as their traditionally taught colleagues. They are better equipped to deal with real clinical situations, better communicators and more able to carry the skills on to lifelong learning (vital for all doctors owing to the speed of advances in the medical world).

Whether you like it or not, many universities in the UK have adopted, or are in the process of adopting, PBL into their courses, either in part or wholeheartedly for the full 5 years. Be aware of this change and be able to express a sensible opinion on the topic if asked at interview. It would be advisable to discuss this type of course with both tutors and students from the practising universities. This is a particularly popular method of teaching the graduate courses.

Universities offering this type of course include Liverpool, Manchester, Glasgow, Queen Mary, Peninsula, Sheffield, Keele, Hull and York, Barts and East Anglia.

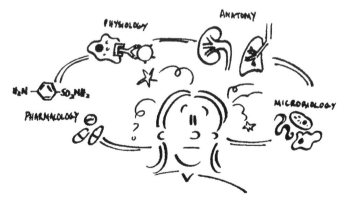

The medical curriculum

10.7 Examinations and assessments

If you have had little experience of exams up until now, then things are about to change. We have mentioned a few of the advantages of being a medical student but by far the biggest disadvantage is the so-called working week and the number of examinations over the 5 years. When you arrive at university, some of your friends in hall may be enrolled on courses where their working week is only 14 hours. Unfortunately, as a medic, you will have a week consisting of 9 to 5 every weekday (and at some places possibly even Saturday mornings!). Your friends will, of course, have exams and probably more course work, so it is not all doom and gloom. Starting at medical school may well introduce you to different types of examination formats.

The true/false exam

This is a slight variation on the multiple choice exam that you will have been familiar with following A levels. It usually involves a stem question followed by several statements. All questions have to be answered and the statement given is either true or false (not exactly rocket science). The problem is that if you answer incorrectly, then you are deducted a point, so-called negative marking. There is therefore an option to abstain (don't know). Not all universities use the negative marking system and some may use the multiple choice format rather than true/false. Another similar format is 'best of five' – there is a stem for the question and then you have to pick the answer from five options.

The short-answer exam and essay exam

This is self-explanatory. It usually requires a bit more studying than the true/false exam.

Viva voce exam

This is an oral exam where you will be questioned on a topic by one or two examiners. These normally last for around 15 minutes. The topics can include physiology and pharmacology. Anatomy is also examined in this way but often will involve the examiners using pro-sections (a dissected part of the body) to focus the discussion.

Practical session

Occasionally some subjects may be examined from a slightly more practical perspective. Examples include histology, where various slides will be shown under microscopes; pathology, where various frozen sections could be presented; and physiology, where you may be required to demonstrate an experiment.

Clinical skills

Traditionally, clinical skills were not really assessed during the early part of university. This has changed with the integrated courses and clinical-type examination formats are often used even in the first year. These can take the format of OSCE (Objective Structured Clinical Examination) and OSLER (Objective Structured Long Examination Record) assessments. It may be necessary to demonstrate practical skills and patient management but obviously to a lesser ability than would be expected in more senior years. These assessment methods are discussed in detail in Chapter 11.

Other types of assessment

During term time some colleges expect essays to be written following small group tutorials, and practical experiment write-ups to be completed, and this may form part of an assessment, but may not count towards your final exams.

10.8 The intercalated degree

This is dealt with in more detail in Chapter 12. It is important to be aware that at some institutions this degree is included as part of the preclinical years so students will obtain a degree at the end of their third year. Most other universities will allow a certain number of students to defer the start of their clinical years by studying for a degree during a further year following their preclinical. At Cambridge and Oxford, the intercalated degree is compulsory and can be taken in a non-medical specialty.

10.9 Summary

It is not so much the difficulty of the work that some students struggle with at university, but more the sheer volume of information required to learn. It is essential not to get too far behind with your work as it will be difficult to catch up. If you have not done biology at A level, some universities will provide some extra tutorials but in our experience it made no difference to students' success at exams. Whichever course is taught, you will be required to spend a significant amount of time for personal study. Reviewing the university prospectuses is essential as the courses still vary with regard to the amount of PBL and the amount of clinical exposure in the first 2 years. Make the most of the clinical time, as it can be very rewarding. Try not to worry too much about the assessments and just take each step at a time – you no doubt remember thinking A levels would be impossible while you were studying for GCSEs, but you got through them!

PERSONAL VIEW   *Alice Gallen*

Who would you regard as being the most important doctor in the last 100 years? This was a question I was asked in three of my four interviews. There had been a public vote on TV that year looking for the top 100 people in the last 100 years – medical schools like to keep interviews topical. Often the questions they ask do not have a right answer.

Taking a gap year was one of the best decisions I have made. I used the time to work in a variety of different jobs and travel. The confidence and life experience I gained from this year helped enormously with the transition to university life. I coped a lot better than I would have done a year earlier.

After filling me up with huge amounts of ice-cream, my real parents left me to go find my new medic parent. My medic 'dad' was a second-year medical student who whisked me off to the medical student bar to welcome me into the medic family. My medic dad was there for the next year to ask questions and just be a friendly face around university.

The first week at medical school seemed to be designed to put people off the whole idea of medicine, at least those who could be put off. We were shown a fictional film of a woman dying of cancer, her treatment and her view of the way she was treated in hospital. We were terrified by the final-year students who came in to quiz us on blood pressure, and in their own humorous ways welcome us to medical school. We also visited the dissection room, a hot smelly room of 30 dead bodies, where at least one person fainted.

It turned out life at medical school was brilliant. Part of the fun was the challenge of the amount of work to do while keeping up with the sporting and social life; life was very busy. The lecture theatre is not the only place where there was a lot to learn. The concept of 'secret working' was entirely new to me. Fellow students would brag about how little work they had done and how little they knew but then would always be the ones to pass and even get merits in the exams. This competitive aspect underlies medical school all the way through. The wish to appear as though you are so intelligent that you do not need to work for knowledge to miraculously appear in your brain is what many medical students aim for. In fact, while some people may need to do a bit more work than others, everyone has to work hard to get through medical school.

My best marks were the modules where I kept my folder organized and worked with a friend, learning a few topics each and then teaching and testing each other. The competitiveness can be a good motivator to work hard, but there is no quota for passing or failing students so it should not stop you helping each other. The reality is that teamwork is a big part of being a doctor and practising this early can help with making friends and passing exams.

Joining the medics rowing team was a big part of my first 2 years at medical school. The team were there to share the experience of the cold rowing sessions on the river, the gossip from sports night in the medic bar and the worries about exams. This also had the advantage of meeting people from all years of medical school, who were able to give tips and some idea about what was involved in the years ahead. There is every possible type of club at university; the biggest decision is which one you will join! They all have the same benefits of meeting people, making sure life does not revolve around exams, and giving you extra skills to put on your CV.

It is compulsory at my university to take a year out and do an intercalated BSc. I took the unusual opportunity to experience a different university for the year and studied sport and exercise science at Loughborough, the course I had wanted to do before I decided on medicine. This was a wonderful year with the excitement of meeting new people and learning a lot about health rather than disease. The main advantage was the dissertation project, which introduced me to the world of research. My project was presented at an international conference and ultimately helped me to be successful in getting the job I wanted, which has a research aspect to it.

Overall, the first 2 years are hard, with a lot of information to learn without really feeling like you are actually going to be a doctor. However, it is a time when you can really enjoy the extracurricular side of university life and completion of these years is the gateway to the clinical years, which is where the fun really begins!

Chapter 11 **The medical course: later years**

You have survived all the lectures, dissection, practical sessions and, more importantly, numerous exams; now it is time to embark on life as a full-time clinical student. It is the time to put all the theory into practice and start to get a feel for what being a doctor is really like; life can change quite dramatically at this time. Many of the students with whom you started at university will have graduated at the end of the third year, going to 'real jobs' and possibly earning considerable amounts of money; however, as a clinical student, your debts will increase further. This is not helped by the fact that holidays become scarce and it is time to buy a new wardrobe (not literally) – it is important as a clinical student to look and act the part. It is time to leave the jeans and T-shirts behind and completely revamp your wardrobe collection with smart outfits. Although still a student, you have a responsibility as a medic to dress and act in a professional and appropriate way. This means ironed clothes (possibly quite a shock for some people) and smart outfits.

There may be times as a student on the wards when you feel more in the way rather than actually being useful. The staff in a hospital will nearly always be busy and it is easy to shy away and try not to be a nuisance. This is not to be recommended. Medical students can play a very helpful role in clinical practice. Often you will be the first person to meet a patient when they are admitted. The impression you give initially will represent the hospital and the other staff. As a student you will often have more time to spend with the patients and through this be able to build a trust. Many of the health professionals who will see the patient later will not have the time to sit and listen as much. For this reason it is possible that you may find out information that the doctors have not elicited, and you can also follow the patient's admission more closely. Whether in third year, fourth year or even

The Essential Guide to Becoming a Doctor, 3rd edition. © Adrian Blundell,
Richard Harrison and Benjamin Turney. Published 2011 by Blackwell Publishing Ltd.

earlier, the first real patient contact can be quite daunting but this can be quickly overcome by getting stuck in.

11.1 Ward etiquette

It is essential to dress and act in a manner befitting a future doctor whenever in the clinical environment; an identification badge is essential. When arriving at a new clinical attachment, whether in the hospital or community, make yourself known to the reception and nursing staff. Check that they don't mind you being there and ask them if any specific measures need to be taken before going to see patients. In some cases it is necessary to wear gloves and gowns. You must wash or sterilize your hands with alcohol gel before and after patient contact and when entering and leaving wards. A student will normally be attached to a particular ward for a certain time, so it is worth orientating yourself early on. When approaching patients, always introduce yourself and ask their permission before asking questions or examining them. Remember that patients will often be more scared than you are by being in hospital and for this reason you should explain clearly your examination routines or any practical procedures. In some circumstances, you may have to ask a colleague or other member of staff to act as a chaperone – if in any doubt, do not examine a patient on your own. As well as learning the skills of talking to and examining patients, you will learn practical procedures, such as taking blood. Any such procedure must be done under the supervision of a doctor in the early days – again, if in doubt, always ask a senior.

11.2 The introductory course

Before commencing the clinical course, most students embark upon an introductory lecture course. This will include presentations on:
• taking a history from a patient
• communication skills
• basic examination routines
• management of common medical and surgical conditions.
It is not possible to make this completely comprehensive within the first week – it is merely an introduction and most students will have had some experience of these concepts earlier. Taking a history is one of the main skills to be learnt initially. Doctors in all specialties use this skill, although some to a greater extent. It is the art of asking patients questions in order to determine what is wrong with them (the *diagnosis*). Despite the wide variety of expensive tests available, it is often possible to make a diagnosis after asking

such a history. Following on from the history, doctors tend to perform an examination. Students will learn how to perform the examination routines for various systems. It is not possible to become proficient in these new skills within the first week but the lectures are aimed at guiding a student in the right direction. There is no substitute for actually talking to and examining as many patients as possible. A student can be shown an examination routine a thousand times in the lecture theatre but until it is carried out personally, the skill will not be learnt. Prior to examining patients it is quite normal for medical students to practise on each other.

11.3 Clinical firms

The clinical years are divided into various specialty blocks; the idea is to give you experience in most of the common specialties. Generally speaking, the more fundamental the specialty, the more time you spend studying it, but the length of each block will vary depending on the university. Traditionally, a group of medical students would be attached to one particular firm – this term refers to a group of doctors of varying levels (see Chapter 15). With the advent of shift working and modernizing medical careers, we have unfortunately lost this firm structure and this has had a direct effect on not only junior doctors but also medical students. This means a lack of continuity in teaching and often the loss of feeling part of a team. It is sometimes even difficult to get portfolios and log books signed by senior clinicians as often you have spent little time with them. One small advantage is that you get to experience teaching from a wider range of clinicians.

The clinical years normally commence with an introduction to medicine and surgery (junior medicine and junior surgery). During the rest of the clinical years specialties covered will include accident and emergency, anaesthetics, dermatology, ear, nose and throat (ENT), general practice, healthcare of the elderly, obstetrics, gynaecology, ophthalmology, orthopaedics, paediatrics, psychiatry and rheumatology. Increasingly, student-chosen modules are offered at some stage during the clinical years (see later section) and, of course, there is the opportunity to study medicine abroad during the elective. The majority of the fifth year concentrates on revisiting medicine and surgery at a higher level. The medicine and surgery courses cover the vast majority of the specialties under this umbrella (see the individual chapters on training in general medicine and surgery for more information on the choices). Of course, exams once again feature highly in the timetable. Please remember that the medical schools vary considerably in the timing and length of the different attachments, so check with individual institutions.

The clinical curriculum

- Accident and emergency
- Anaesthetics
- Dermatology
- Ear, nose and throat
- Elective
- General practice
- Healthcare of the elderly (geriatrics)
- Medicine
- Obstetrics and gynaecology
- Ophthalmology
- Orthopaedics
- Paediatrics
- Pathology
- Psychiatry
- Radiology
- Rheumatology
- Student-chosen modules
- Surgery

During your clinical years, you may well spend time at other hospitals around your local region. This is to ensure you experience different hospital environments (teaching versus district general) and also to prevent overcrowding: there is just not enough room in the main hospital for all the students at one time. In some instances the attachments can be 12 weeks long and up to 75 miles away. Accommodation will usually be provided by these hospitals but some people buy cars or commute and continue to live in the same place. This can be very difficult to do, especially if finances are tight, so bear it in mind for your budget.

11.4 An average week

The weekly timetables will depend on the current attachment but in general will follow a pattern. The focus of teaching will be on small group tutorials rather than large lectures, although there may be some sessions where you get together as a whole year for central themes. Many of the tutorials will now be around the bedside, learning clinical skills and practical procedures, knowledge that can be reinforced using the clinical skills and simulator laboratories. There will be timetabled teaching sessions with the more senior doctors and these could be topic or skills based. It is necessary to see patients and 'clerk' them (i.e. take a history and perform an examination), to then present to the consultants during their ward rounds. Ad hoc teaching sessions are often as useful and can be given by the more junior staff or other healthcare professionals. Of course you need to be around on the ward for these to occur – in general the staff are too busy to be trying to track the whereabouts of the students if an opportunity for a practical procedure or interesting patient appears, so it is essential to be enthusiastic. During each attachment the relevant pathology and radiology will be taught by experts in these fields in other tutorials. Other sessions will be spent in outpatient clinics or watching procedures and operations. Not all sessions of the timetable will be structured and there will be time to spend on the wards seeing patients and improving clinical skills. It is useful during this time to see the general everyday running of the wards or GP surgeries. Attend the admissions wards, preferably when your consultant is the admitting doctor, and see the patients as they come into the hospital (see section 11.6). Often the most important members of the team will be the junior doctors so tag along with them at free times. They often know where the interesting patients are and will appreciate your help with procedures such as taking blood – oh, and they can point you in the direction of the best coffee and also the doctors' mess. Our advice: be around, be enthusiastic and get involved – you will get much more out of the attachments. It is generally much easier to shy away, and to be honest this will not necessarily be noticed by medical staff, until the exams, when it is too late. Remember keen students get more teaching.

11.5 The clinical attachments

Medicine and surgery (see also Chapters 20 and 21)

Medicine and surgery are the longest components of the clinical course, and there are usually two attachments for each, junior medicine and surgery and senior medicine and surgery. The attachments can be 8–12 weeks long for each. You will spend time attached to a particular team of doctors who will supervise and teach you. There will be opportunities to see and assess patients, practise examinations, and learn clinical skills such as taking blood, resuscitation and other minor procedures. General medicine is also known as internal medicine and is discussed in more detail in Chapter 20. You will spend time on the wards, in the outpatients department and, when studying surgery, in the operating theatre where there is the chance to assist with the operation itself. During surgery attachments many students spend the odd week learning about anaesthetics – this can be good fun and usually results in the acquisition of some useful clinical skills, ranging from insertion of a cannula (a drip) to intubation of patients. Division into medicine and surgery blocks occurs at most medical schools, although some of the newer courses run 'linked blocks', for example respiratory medicine is linked with thoracic surgery. This is not necessarily a better system but does emphasize the multidisciplinary nature of the work as discussed previously.

Obstetrics and gynaecology

Generally, you will spend around 8 weeks in this attachment, and your time will be split between the two areas. In obstetrics, you will spend time in antenatal clinics, seeing and assessing pregnant women, and then spend time in the delivery suite helping deliver babies. This can be quite a nerve-wracking time, but do not worry, you will be closely supervised. You will also spend some time in theatre assisting with Caesarean sections. Gynaecology means time in outpatients and in theatre observing operations such as a hysterectomy.

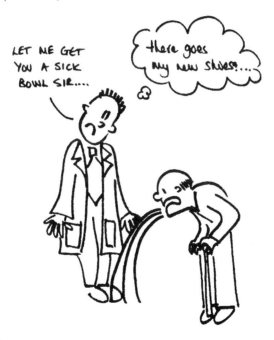

The clinical years

Paediatrics

Although it is obviously distressing seeing poorly children, most students look forward to this attachment. It involves developing different skills as the patients are often not able to give a history and it can be difficult to examine them. There is often time to be spent not only with the children but also with their playstation or other toys. It can be a difficult subject area because of the vast array of diseases that babies and children can develop. Emotions are often high and caring for and communicating with the parents is also essential.

General practice (see also Chapter 19)

The time allocated for this specialty at most universities does not correlate with the fact that the majority of graduates become GPs. Traditionally, most students were only offered a small number of weeks to experience medicine at the community level. This has changed over the last few years and many students now find themselves allocated to a local GP surgery early in their course. This allows several visits over the 5 years and gives some continuity and experience of a very different kind of medicine. After all, spending so much time in the hospital, one can start to think that all patients are unwell and require emergency treatment. This is also a time when teaching is often on a one-to-one basis and a medical student may have their own list of patients to see. During this time it is also possible to spend time with other members of the surgery, for example district nurses and community physiotherapists. The emphasis on community care will increase over the next few years as the government moves more services out of the large acute hospitals. GP attachments should really be longer as it can be a very different kind of medicine, with much less availability of instant investigations. Most students enjoy the courses where regular visits to the same surgery are organized as they appreciate the experience of continuity.

Other attachments

The attachments mentioned above tend to be the longest. The time allocated to each of the other parts of the clinical spectrum will vary depending on the university. Although the specialties are divided at medical school, the reality is that there is great overlap and doctors often have joint meetings (multidisciplinary meetings or MDTs). For example, a patient with lung cancer would be discussed and seen at a clinic which could have doctors and other healthcare professionals from respiratory medicine, oncology, palliative care, radiology, pathology and thoracic surgery; there is great emphasis on team-working. In this way expertise can be offered and a management plan devised. During the clinical years some subjects (e.g. radiology and pathology) will not have an allocated time but will be covered on each attachment so that, for example, the pathology and radiology of gynaecology will be studied during that attachment.

The clinical years offer an insight into the reality of becoming and working as a doctor. The attachments should be enjoyable but at the same time can be hard work. Most will have formal examinations, although some may use course work as an assessment.

11.6 On-call

Another essential element of the clinical years is to spend time 'on-call', preferably with members of your team. During this time it is possible to clerk (take a history and examine) many of the patients, even before the doctors have seen them. In this way a student doctor can get used to presenting the patient's history and examination findings to the more senior members of the team and also start considering management plans. It is then possible to follow the patient from admission to discharge. If any of the patients require surgery or other procedures, then it is useful to attend and help at these.

11.7 Examinations and assessments

All the specialties during your clinical years will be assessed in one way or another. The timing of these will vary with each medical school. The more traditional universities favour the concept of finals. This refers to a set of examinations at the end of fifth year, which test knowledge on all the subjects studied during the clinical years. The more modern courses involve assessments at the end of blocks of subjects. This has the advantage of not revising such a huge number of subjects at the end of the course but does require more regular work throughout the clinical years. The type of examinations and assessments include those introduced in the preclinical years and also involve more practical-based tests.

OSCE/ISCE (Objective/Integrated Structured Clinical Examination)

This involves a series of stations lasting a few minutes each, where various clinical skills will be tested. This could include patient examination, taking a history, describing X-rays or interpreting clinical data. These types of exams have been shown to be fairer because each candidate has the same questions and examiner.

OSLER (Objective Structured Long Examination Record)

This assessment has replaced the older style long case exam, although is only used at a small number of medical schools. It involves a student spending a set amount of time (usually about 45 minutes) with a patient during which the student takes a history and performs a relevant examination. Following this, the student will be joined by the examiner who will ask questions about the case, which will include clinical findings, diagnosis and management. The examiners will also ask the patient's opinion of the student doctor.

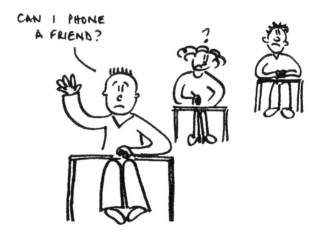

Medical examinations

Short cases

This involves a candidate seeing several cases while being accompanied by an examiner. It may involve examination of certain systems or good use of observational powers, while being questioned.

Log books and portfolios

Many of these attachments use log books as a way of assessing progression through the course. These will list objectives and then have sections to be filled in listing various practical and learning experiences that should be gained, and which need to be signed by your teachers. Not all students like the log book approach as it seems like a signature-obtaining game. It should be noted that the log books are to be used as a guide and contain the bare minimum required by a student to complete the attachment.

11.8 Student-chosen modules

This concept has been introduced over the last few years and is now commonplace in the clinical curriculum. During the clinical years a student spends one or two clinical attachments studying a topic of their choice. This can mean further general training, in paediatrics for example, or choosing a more specialist subject which you may not experience otherwise, for example forensic medicine. The other advantage of this attachment is that there may well be no written examinations, although some course work is usually expected. If you already have an idea of your chosen specialty once you qualify, then this is a perfect opportunity to determine if your decision is correct. Bear in mind it will not be possible for every student to get their first choice. Some universities also arrange exchange programmes abroad; the options will then be endless, although language may be a barrier. Student-selected components now form a significant proportion of the curriculum time at some medical schools, up to 20% in some instances.

11.9 The elective (see Chapter 12)

OK, so you have worked hard for the last 4 or 5 years and over the clinical years there has been little evidence of holidays. There is one part of the clinical curriculum that should be eagerly awaited – the elective. So let's get this straight: as part of your course, you are allowed to spend up to 2 months travelling the world and possibly even get funding. Well that is not exactly true (for most at any rate!).

11.10 The shadowing weeks

Towards the end of your training, most universities now provide a shadowing period. This will occur at the end of the course, before commencing your Foundation year 1 post and is an opportunity to 'shadow' the junior doctor that you will be replacing later in the year. This period may be split with some lecture-based material, for example the logistics of completing death certificates and reporting deaths to the coroner, but the majority of the time will be spent in the clinical environment. This will give you the opportunity to get to know a little about the hospital where you will be starting. This is important because all hospitals differ slightly in their arrangements, for example ordering of tests. It should help you settle into what will become your new home for the next few months. It would be unwise to miss any of this time. It is your last chance to get up to speed with managing patients and procedures with maximal support from the doctors and other staff. If you feel that there are any weaknesses in the skills that you should have gained, now is the time to correct them.

11.11 Graduation

So, you have finally made it. Five years of hard work (and hopefully considerable fun) are now behind you. It is time to look forward to your chosen career and the success that this will bring. Before this, it is time for some well-earned celebrating. At the end of the academic year is the formal graduation ceremony. Now is the time for parents and loved ones to watch their children receive their graduation certificates in full gown and mortar board. They will fully appreciate the time, effort and financial support that has been necessary over the preceding 5 years. The culmination of the 5 years will be the graduation ball. No doubt, a committee will have volunteered early during the fifth year to arrange this grand event. Fundraising may actually have started many years earlier. You will only ever experience one medical graduation ball, so enjoy it!

11.12 Summary

Most students spend the early years at medical school looking forward to the clinical attachments; it is when you start learning about the real way in which doctors work and seems far more relevant to your future career than the time spent in the lecture theatre learning the Krebs cycle for the third time! The downside includes the reduction in university holidays and the increasing expense, for example smart clothes, transport to and from hospitals, and further books and equipment. It can also be far more daunting than the early years, having to communicate with patients and perform intimate examinations. A minority of students also discover that the sight of blood and being around sick patients is not for them and leave to pursue other careers. In general most students graduate from medical school on the first attempt and then gain provisional registration with the GMC to embark on their Foundation programme.

PERSONAL VIEW   *Jamie Read*

My first day on the wards as a 'clinical years' medical student was met with mixed emotions; excitement that I seemed another step closer to the career that I had chosen to pursue, anxiety at the dreaded teaching ward rounds which seemed scarred into the memory of most doctors in the hospital, and shock at just how ill some patients were.

Initially, everything seemed foreign; I couldn't work out who was who or where I needed to be at certain times and no one seemed to have any time to sit down with me and explain anything. As a result I returned home after my first day utterly exhausted and overwhelmed by the whole experience. That first day is somewhat a rite of passage for medical students and, trust me, things do get better! Once I had been introduced to my consultant and the rest of the team, I was able to start making the ward I was attached to feel more like my own. I made sure I introduced myself to all the staff on the ward (never underestimate how important everyone on the ward can be when you are having a bad day) and I set about trying to see as many patients as possible. This can be quite daunting but was made considerably easier by stories from other students that patients are generally very happy to see you and that they want to help you learn. Often taking the time to speak to them helps to break the boredom of being confined to a hospital bed so in many cases they are glad to see you. It really can help to have developed your small talk for those slightly uncomfortable introductions, especially as there are only so many times that you can joke about curtains being sound-proof when the reality is that what the patient is saying to you can be heard by every other person on the ward!

Having survived the first couple of weeks, one of the real challenges that I found was balancing time in the hospital and time spent looking up all the things that had happened that I didn't understand; to begin with there is rather a lot to look up. This does mean that you'll have to put your organizational skills to good use and there are times when you will wish that you had a clone when your consultant wants you to be in one place, the medical school in another and that society you joined in first year is having a social at the same time. Again, I found that this became much easier with time and also I learnt to say no; after all there are only so many endoscopies you can watch before you can't learn any more and hence finding something else to do is generally a good idea.

Another change I found was that entering my clinical years almost felt like I had stopped being a student and more like I had a job; I suddenly had more responsibility, was expected to dress smartly and had scheduled activities throughout the day which did not include just walking to university and sitting through a lecture. While this can feel strange at first it does pose its own set of opportunities. As a clinical years medical student you suddenly become useful. You help out with ward jobs and it allowed me to put all the knowledge that I acquired in year 1 and 2 into practice. There is also a lot to be said for being in the right place at the right time and if you put the hours in then the opportunities can be fairly endless. I've had the opportunity to practise venepuncture, cannulation, intubate patients, relieve a tension pneumothorax, assist in theatres and speak to some very interesting patients, each of whom has a life history that can be quite inspirational. To make the most of these opportunities it pays to be pushy – people will not always offer

(continued)

(*Continued*)

you opportunities, you need to ask for them. This can be hard as I often felt I was in the way; these worries are unfounded though and it's important to remember that you are an integral part of the team who needs to be given opportunities as much as anyone else – don't be afraid of reminding people of this!

Unfortunately, this sudden and significant change between a preclinical and clinical medical student can be hard to appreciate by friends at university who are not medics. A lot of my friends didn't quite seem to understand what my day-to-day work as a student involved; they were used to going to lectures and going home to watch daytime TV rather than spending long days trying to gain knowledge and skills in the hospital. Discussing my day suddenly seemed very foreign to them and this tends to draw you even closer to the people who you are studying with. This can be great, but I would definitely recommend developing other interests outside medicine to maintain your sanity.

Being a clinical years medical student is a great opportunity and one that I have really enjoyed. I have learnt a huge amount and got to learn some really useful clinical skills and it's made me feel very prepared to be a junior doctor. The most important thing to say is, don't give up; sometimes it can feel hard but the good days far outnumber the bad and I have no regrets about my career choice.

Good luck!

Chapter 12 **The intercalated degree**

To intercalate means to insert among others. The intercalated degree is one that you take during study for another. The prime purpose of medical school is to graduate as a Bachelor of Medicine and a Bachelor of Surgery (these have various abbreviations depending on the university attended, e.g. BM BS, MB BS, MB BChir). During study for this primary degree, it is often possible to carry out some research towards an extra degree, the *intercalated degree*. These vary in form: some are carried out within the 5-year medical degree course while others require extra time – some an extra 6 months, some an extra year. Most allow you to graduate as a Bachelor of Science (BSc), but there are variations on a theme.

12.1 Popularity

One-third of medical students in the UK study for an intercalated degree during their undergraduate course, but the proportion varies according to the medical school. At some schools, the opportunity to take this additional degree depends on performance in the first couple of years, while at others it is an integral part of the curriculum.

12.2 The choices

There is little consistency between the types of degree offered by the different medical schools and although some traditionally have been regarded as being better, in reality they have the same benefit. The majority of medical schools offer a BSc or a BMedSci. Occasionally the degree gained is a BA,

The Essential Guide to Becoming a Doctor, 3rd edition. © Adrian Blundell,
Richard Harrison and Benjamin Turney. Published 2011 by Blackwell Publishing Ltd.

a Bachelor of Arts degree, which is bit of a paradox considering that most medical students are very science orientated. An uncommon option offered is an integrated PhD. This may be done as a separate intercalated 3-year degree between preclinical and clinical years or sometimes is integrated into an extended 5-year clinical course (e.g. at Cambridge).

- Compulsory BSc: Imperial College, London, St Andrews.
- Optional BSc: available at most medical schools.
- BMedSci within the 5-year course: Nottingham.
- BMedSci as an extra year: Sheffield.
- BA: Oxford and Cambridge.
- PhD: selected universities.

12.3 Which subjects are available?

The subjects are usually basic science orientated, the reason being that the departments available to the medical school for these projects are those teaching the basic medical sciences during the preclinical years. There are other options depending on the university and sometimes it is even possible to study at a different establishment.

Possible intercalated subjects

- Anatomy
- Cell biology
- Epidemiology
- History of medicine
- Medical biochemistry
- Medical law
- Medical microbiology
- Neuroscience
- Pharmacology
- Physiology
- Psychology
- Public health

12.4 The objectives

The main principle behind the intercalated degree is to develop the ability to evaluate research critically and understand the principles underlying its methodology, skills necessary for lifelong medical learning and practice. The best way of acquiring these analytical skills is by conducting in-depth research oneself. Also, with the deepening recruitment crisis in academic medicine, encouraging those contemplating such a career should be a priority. Thirdly, allowing medics to interact with a new and diverse peer group can broaden horizons and offer fresh perspectives on the learning process. This research period offers time to study a selected area of biomedical technology in depth, usually by means of lectures and a research project. It is hoped a student will gain:

- a greater depth of knowledge of some area of medical science that underpins modern medicine;
- the ability to critically evaluate previous and current research, the biomedical literature and data;
- the ability to communicate scientific information in a variety of formats;
- research skills enabling design, execution, interpretation and reporting of experiments in an area of biomedical sciences.

The experience brings some of the scientific theory learnt in the first couple of years of medical school to relevance, for example learning what PCR and Western blotting really are, developing good computing skills such as database management, presentation skills, journal article searching, and familiarity with statistics.

There is also a recreational element to the additional year, with more free time. This time can be spent with the many medical societies; it gives an additional extra summer with the opportunity to travel the world; and can also provide extra maturity, making you ready for the demanding clinical years.

12.5 The benefits

Educationally

If you wish to pursue an academic career, then an intercalated degree is sensible, as it will allow you to develop research skills, think critically, study the scientific basis of medical sciences, and prove to others that you are academically motivated. If you really do want to work in a laboratory later in life, the experience gained during the year could be invaluable. Currently, some specialties do require that people have higher degrees, and the intercalated degree will be useful for applying for those positions. Being taught by scientific members of staff and having the opportunity to experience the excitement and challenges of science will certainly be a change from sitting in the medical school lecture theatres.

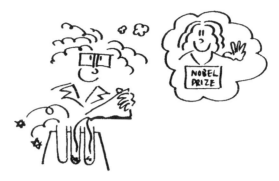

The intercalated degree

Clinically

There does not seem to be a correlation between undertaking an interca-lated degree and clinical excellence. Will it help you get the best jobs when training as a junior doctor? Possibly – there is no doubt that the extra degree will look good on paper, but it is uncertain as to how much influence this would have on your chances of being shortlisted. Some of the best consult-ants in the country do not have an intercalated degree, indeed some of them have no formal academic research qualifications at all. Having said this, the competitive areas of medicine often use academic criteria to discriminate candidates and further higher degrees (e.g. MSc, MD, PhD) can be required, and undergraduate degrees can help with securing these at a later date. Remember that, following qualification, most junior doctors' CVs are very similar, so anything that can make you stand out will be useful.

Leaving medicine

If you decide that medicine is not for you, then having a BSc or BMedSci on the CV will look good and gives you the opportunity to get out of medicine after 3 years with a recognized science degree.

12.6 The downside

Taking additional time to undertake the intercalated degree costs in terms of time and money. The cost of studying is not inconsiderable and has increased in recent years due to tuition fees and higher living costs. The additional year of study will cost thousands of pounds. Occasionally fund-ing is available, but this is usually only available to those who are undertak-ing higher degrees.

12.7 Summary

The best way to decide whether to study for a further degree is to weigh up the pros and cons, mainly the educational benefits versus the financial costs. One possible way round the financial cost is to plump for Nottingham – they offer a BMedSci without an additional year. Other options include completing the medical course and then applying for an academic foundation programme or taking time out later on, during your career path, to study for a higher degree (MSc, MD, PhD).

PERSONAL VIEW   *Rick Harrison*

My decision to study for an intercalated degree really started before I applied to medical school. I thought it sounded like a good idea and specifically applied to medical schools which offered the intercalated degree as part of the course. I was accepted at and chose to attend Nottingham University, which offers a BMedSci degree as part of the 5-year course. This basically means that your preclinical and clinical time is compressed slightly and your period of research is done during the third year. It means you have to work harder than students at other medical schools, but you 'save' a year overall.

Although the intercalated degree is 'built in' at Nottingham, as with most medical schools there was a broad choice of departments and subjects to study, for example pharmacology, physiology and anatomy. I chose the Department of Anatomy as I thought this was most relevant to what I thought I wanted to do in the future, which was surgery.

I was allocated a supervisor who I met with on most days and he set me the research task. I had to grow cultured cells in a laboratory in different conditions to see how well they could grow. I won't blind you with the science – although it sounds hi-tech, all the procedures were taught to me. Friends in different departments were generally working on a small part of a large ongoing project. Some were helping with clinical trials (those conducted on patients), some were working in the lab, while others were helping to write software programs. Some students even devised their own projects.

Although hard work during the day, there were no lectures to study for or tutorials to prepare for, which left the evenings free for sport or other activities. This was a pleasant break from lots of library work, which I knew would be restarting at the end of the year.

(continued)

(Continued)

The research project lasted for around 8 months and at the end of this I had to complete a dissertation of around 15 000 words, which formed the basis of the assessment for the degree. This dissertation was examined with a viva exam, which was genuinely quite frightening. I was awarded a 2:1 degree which I was very pleased with.

Although hard work, I think the experience was worthwhile; medical practice is based around research and 'evidence', and knowing how that knowledge is compiled can be very useful. Good luck if you choose to do one!

Chapter 13 **The elective**

This will, without doubt, be one of the most memorable elements of your life at medical school. The medical elective is a period in the medical curriculum lasting between 8 and 12 weeks (depending on the individual medical school) when you are given the freedom to choose what and where you want to study. You are allowed to go to any medical establishment in the world! The major difficulties are in choosing where to go and how to afford it. Different medical schools put the elective in different places in the curriculum. It is invariably in the final 2 years of the course after you have at least some clinical training.

13.1 The official bit

The purpose of the elective is to allow you to explore in detail a field of medicine that you find of particular interest or an area that you felt was inadequately covered in the medical curriculum. It is included because it allows an opportunity to experience medicine in a different social, cultural, economic and scientific environment. Some medical students with a real interest in a subject go to a renowned centre of excellence in that subject to make contacts and develop that all-important CV.

Medical schools are aware that 22 year olds given 2–3 months off might take an opportunity to have a rather good long holiday. It is therefore compulsory to write a report of what you have done and, at some universities, return a signed form from the hospital where you visited, to certify that you spent time where you said you were going to work.

13.2 The unofficial bit

Traditionally, medical students have used the elective as a once in a lifetime opportunity to travel to far-flung places where the sun shines all day long

The Essential Guide to Becoming a Doctor, 3rd edition. © Adrian Blundell,
Richard Harrison and Benjamin Turney. Published 2011 by Blackwell Publishing Ltd.

and to have adventures that become the stuff of legend and of stories and anecdotes for the rest of their medical careers – 'I was in a bar in the remotest of the Pacific islands when. . .'

Most hospitals that have had medical students (especially those in traditional elective hotspots) know the score and will happily do a deal where you do so many days a week or a block of weeks to get things signed and enough information to write a report and then allow you time for travel. In this way it is possible to combine the educational and the enjoyable and keep everyone happy!

13.3 How do you choose where to go on elective?

Choosing an elective is extremely difficult. There are some fundamental questions that you need to ask yourself before you make up your mind.

What do I want to get out of my elective?

Do you want a valuable educational experience? Some people want to go to a centre of excellence for a particular discipline. If you are considering a career in a particular field, it may allow you to explore this further and make some contacts for the future. This gives you an opportunity at an early stage to assess whether you really think that a particular area of medicine is for you or not. This sort of elective is more difficult to organize and can be a disappointment if things don't quite work out as you want.

If you primarily want a holiday, there are lots of places that are very used to having elective students and will give you advice about where to go to explore when you get there.

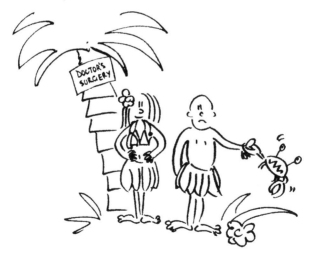

What do I want to get out of my elective?

What sort of weather do I want?

Do you want sunshine or snow? Depending on the time of year when your elective appears in the curriculum, you need to decide which part of the world you want to be in. If your elective is in the autumn/winter and you want sun, then think of the southern hemisphere.

Developed or developing country?

This is a fundamental question. The practice of medicine in developing countries varies dramatically from that in the UK. The living conditions and the diseases are very different and you will see things that you may never see in the UK. Also the treatments are different and these are limited by availability of equipment, drugs and medical and nursing staff. In the past medical students were allowed to provide all sorts of treatment and surgery in developing countries and often benefited many patients. However, you are still a medical student and as you are not qualified you shouldn't be practising on patients in these parts of the world. There are now strict guidelines regarding what you should and should not do with regard to patient treatment on elective. Despite this you are more likely to be involved in patient care in the developing world than in developed countries.

Working in a developed country allows you to compare how medical care is organized and the good and bad points of an alternative healthcare system. However, you tend not to get as much in the way of experience.

UK is OK!

Of course, you don't have to go abroad to do your elective. It is becoming more common to stay in the UK, for a variety of reasons. Indeed, experience gained in this country can be very useful for gaining contacts for future jobs. There is always the possibility to travel later on in your career and the cost of an elective in the UK is cheaper.

English speaking?

You don't have to go to an English-speaking country. If you have other languages, then the elective is a fantastic opportunity to go and practise your language skills. If you are not very confident with another language, medical conditions and symptoms can be very confusing. The elective may allow you to develop a foreign language, but bear in mind that it is probably better to be in an environment where there is more time to talk to patients and the staff have more time to help you if your knowledge of the language is not great. For example, A&E (accident and emergency) is not a good environment for learning a new language.

Alone or with friends?

You will need to decide whether you want to go in a group or by yourself. There is safety in numbers and it does mean that you can travel with friends and remind each other of the adventures that you experienced together when you are back home. Going as a group is probably a good option if you primarily want a 'relaxing' elective.

Going as an individual will allow you to have more freedom to be who you want to be and it forces you to make more effort to meet new people. It is generally much easier to organize your elective by yourself, especially if you want to go to a specific place in a specific department. Alternatively, you can try to combine it and meet up with friends on the other side of the world after your elective for a bit of travelling.

13.4 Organization

Electives are not easy to organize from scratch. Most medical schools have copies of previous elective reports in the library with contact addresses and tips. Many consultants have colleagues/friends who work around the world. If you have a particular subject interest, then go and talk to the relevant consultants. They may be able to put you in touch with their opposite number in a foreign country. Speak with the students in the year above. Most of them will be pleased to bore you with their elective stories and you might just learn a few handy tips! Most medical schools throughout the world have a website and some have a dedicated section on electives. There are a couple of books available that give general guidance about different electives and what you can expect. However, a personal contact is best, as there is often plenty of bureaucracy involved and if you have a friendly contact at the other end, things are much easier. Most medical schools also hold an annual elective evening, with presentations from those students who went travelling the previous year and various travel firms are invited to have displays.

13.5 Financial limits

How much can you afford? The elective is a one-off experience and it would be a shame to restrict yourself. Funding is very scarce though and will often not be available at all. Many medical schools offer small bursaries of a few hundred pounds but are only able to offer them to a small number of people. If you know what subject area interests you for your future career, there are some Royal College grants and bursaries available.

Having said this, the reality is that you will probably have to fund the majority, if not all, of the elective by yourself. The BMA do offer loans at attractive rates for medical students and many think this a worthwhile thing to do. See Chapter 14 for other funding advice.

13.6 Planning

Whatever you choose you must start to plan early! Some electives are very popular, for example the flying doctors in Australia and trauma electives in the USA. If you are thinking of this sort of thing you need to start writing to the organizers about a year in advance.

Send off several applications. Reply quickly if you accept. Let people know if you decline so they can reallocate to other students. Correspondence takes time even with e-mail and there is plenty to organize other than which hospital you are going to and which consultant you will be with. You will also need to think about accommodation, necessary vaccinations, visas, medical malpractice insurance and personal health insurance.

13.7 Safety on elective

You have a responsibility to keep yourself safe on elective. Most universities can provide a travel pack with basic medical equipment and a few simple drugs (e.g. antibiotics). Remember that HIV has a high prevalence in some countries and that precautions and even avoidance of high-risk procedures is recommended. More information about travelling can be found in Chapter 4.

13.8 Summary

The medical elective is a unique part of the course so make the most of it whatever you decide to do. Remember that organization is the key and for some electives you will need to start preparing 12–18 months in advance.

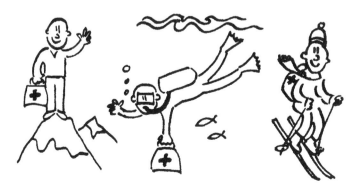

The medical elective is a unique part of the course . . . make the most of it!

PERSONAL VIEW   *Torquil Duncan-Brown*

'Here you are – you're the doctor!' These words were among the first I heard as I arrived on my student elective on the Pacific island of Samoa. It was the senior midwife speaking and she had just deposited a blue, lifeless, 1-minute-old baby into my hands. Was I petrified or exhilarated? I didn't know what to think! Here I was finally being given responsibility after all the years of learning. And what was more, I was in the most idyllic place for a hospital you can imagine. Blue skies, green seas and white beaches only a 2-minute walk away. I had got there via a week in Hawaii and was returning via New Zealand and Hong Kong.

It all needed a little organization and planning, but I had landed myself with such a great opportunity. Not only was I going to a beautiful Pacific island, but the route there enabled me to stop off and explore elsewhere. I spent the first of the 10 weeks away in Hawaii. Travellers were everywhere and I spent the week with a couple a people I met out there tripping around the islands watching sunrises from the top of a mountain, listening to whales swimming with us in the sea and drinking cocktails to the sunsets. The route back gave me the chance to see some friends for a few days in New Zealand and Hong Kong.

The work as a student in the larger of the two hospitals was a little like being at home but with my own clinics to run. When I went to the more isolated of the two islands, I found myself with more responsibility than I could have dreamed of. It all seemed a little daunting. Yet here I was running my own clinics and dealing with anything from chesty babies and children with heart failure to pregnancies and multiple trauma casualties from car accidents. I was just entrusted to get on with it and do the best I could. I took and developed my own X-rays, did my own ward rounds and wrote prescriptions. There was always a doctor on hand to supervise, but it was an invaluable learning time when I got used to the responsibility and the chance to use all that knowledge from the past years, for what felt like the first time outside of exams. And in my spare time I got to see the tourist sites and some lesser-known places to visit on the islands. After work I would walk down to the beach and float around in the sea during the tropical storm, or just relax and watch the incredible sunsets. The locals were so friendly and I became something of a local celebrity when I adopted local dress (a type of sarong) to work in! This was the life.

My elective really was one of the highlights of my student days, and looking back it has provided me with perhaps some of the vital skills for what lay ahead – my house jobs – plenty of responsibility, independence and, more importantly, the ability to unwind from work.

Chapter 14 **Finances**

Four to six years at university doesn't come cheap. The financial help available to a student depends on several factors including parental income, type of course (undergraduate or graduate), location of university and country of birth. Financial support is available for all students entering higher education, although the support differs depending on which of the four home nations you are from. Applications for student finance need to be registered with your individual area, namely Student Finance England, Student Finance Wales, Student Finance Northern Ireland or Student Awards Agency for Scotland. Once you have decided that you will be applying for higher education, it is wise to start looking into the details of financial support available.

14.1 The hard facts: tuition fees

England
For 2010, students studying in England are required to pay tuition fees of up to a maximum of £3225 per year, depending on the course and university.

Northern Ireland
Students starting their course in 2010 will have to contribute up to £3225 per annum to the cost of their university education.

Scotland
Eligible Scottish domiciled (ordinarily living in Scotland) and non-UK EU students studying in Scotland normally apply to the Student Awards Agency for Scotland (SAAS) to have their tuition fees paid. Students from England,

The Essential Guide to Becoming a Doctor, 3rd edition. © Adrian Blundell,
Richard Harrison and Benjamin Turney. Published 2011 by Blackwell Publishing Ltd.

Wales and Northern Ireland starting their medical studies in Scotland in 2010 will be charged the tuition fee set by the institution they have chosen to study at. They will need to apply to their local educational authorities to find out if they are eligible for any financial support.

Wales
From 2010, students studying in Wales are required to pay tuition fees of up to a maximum of £3225 per year. Students ordinarily living in Wales and attending a Welsh university are eligible, regardless of family income, for a yearly £1940 grant paid directly to the place of study towards tuition fees.

14.2 The hard facts: living expenses

On top of the tuition fees are considerable fees for living expenses. The loan companies anticipate that students will require about £4400 a year to cover these costs (more if in London and less if living at home). Many students find it difficult to keep within this budget. Assuming you do keep within this budget, the total cost per year (fees and living costs) will be £7400 per year, which works out at £37 000 for a 5-year course. It could of course be much more.

Student outgoings

- Tuition fees
- Accommodation
- Food
- Bills
- Books/equipment
- Socializing
- Money for holidays
- Car/bike costs
- Room insurance
- Mobile phone
- Clothing
- University societies

14.3 Money management

It is important to organize your finances at the beginning of a term and try to budget for the next few weeks. Student loans are paid into your account at the beginning of term and it is necessary to avoid a false sense of wealth, otherwise you may find yourself overspent halfway through term. Many students who study medicine have affluent parents, so it is important to remember to live within your own means if your financial situation is different. Try to avoid wasting money on too many textbooks or university societies in the first few weeks. It is still possible to make purchases and join clubs later in the term. Hopefully your debt will not be too great after the first 2 years and most students manage with some common sense and knowing about certain sources of available funding.

The cheapest option at university is to live with your parents. This is not to be recommended as it is important to experience life away from home and anyway most students travel to a different city, so commuting is impossible. University accommodation tends to be reasonable value and the rent often covers bills and food. Once you are living away from the halls and colleges, the cost of rent is likely to increase dramatically. For popular shared houses in university towns it is not unusual to be paying around £50–70 per week, although prices can vary considerably. This does not normally include bills or food, although you won't have to pay council tax. Some areas will be more expensive than others, London being a prime example of a very expensive place.

During the clinical years it does become harder to keep your bank balance in the black. This is due to a combination of longer terms and different expenditure. Expenses include the purchase of smart clothes and possibly a car. This is obviously not essential but many of the clinical year attachments will be at other hospitals within the area, so transport is useful. Longer terms means fewer holidays and so most decide against employment and opt for exotic breaks to recover from the strenuous work.

No student should be prevented from going to university because of his or her financial situation. The Government and other organizations have methods to help those less well off. This includes help with the cost of tuition fees and also with loans. Working during a gap year can enable a few pennies to be saved ready for the start of term but most students tend to spend the money they earn during this year on travel before university. The majority of students will need to take out a student loan as a minimum. The following section covers some other sources of available income.

14.4 Main sources of financial help

Other than financial support from your family, there are many ways to find the money to pay for your university career. The main ones are student loans, maintenance grants (for those from households with lower incomes) and awards from the university you attend. There are other separate funds available for disabled students and those with children. There are also other sources of funding such as bank loans.

Student loans

Students can now take loans for both tuition fees and living costs from the Student Loan Company (SLC) (www.slc.co.uk). They attract a very low rate of interest (at inflation levels). This ensures that the value of the loan that is repaid remains the same in real terms as the amount borrowed. Currently, the interest rate is –0.4%, which is good news but not likely to last long! Interest rates have generally averaged around 2% in the last couple of years.

Tuition fees

Eligible full-time undergraduate students do not have to pay tuition fees before they start university or while they are studying; instead eligible students are able to apply for a Student Loan for Fees to cover these costs (currently £3225 per annum). The fees will be paid direct to the university or college on behalf of the student. Students will repay these loans once they have left university and are earning over £15 000. There are no upper age limits imposed for Student Loan for Fees.

Living costs

Student loans are also available to help with living costs. The table below shows the maximum maintenance loans available.

	Living at home	Living away from home outside London	Living away from home in London
Maximum student loan for maintenance	£3838	£4950	£6928
Not income assessed (72%)	£2763	£3564	£4988
Income assessed (about 28%)	£1075	£1386	£1940

The loan is repayable in instalments once you leave your course and start earning more than £15 000 a year. Deductions are usually made direct from your salary (through the PAYE tax system) by your employer in the same way as tax and National Insurance contributions. Repayments are proportionate to your earnings. For example, someone earning £20 000 a year would currently repay £8.65 a week or £37.50 a month. If you stop working or your earnings fall below £15 000, then you don't have to make repayments.

Maintenance grants

In 2009 if your household income is below £25 000, you will be eligible for a non-repayable maintenance grant of £2906 a year. Partial grants are also available for students with an annual household income between £25 001 and £50 200.

Grants from universities and colleges

All universities running medical courses are obliged to provide non-repayable bursaries to students who are receiving the full maintenance grant (£2906). This will be at least £300 a year. Contact your university to see what they are offering.

Other grants

Some students may have specific circumstances warranting further financial help. This may come in the form of grants or allowances. As each situation is unique to the individual, it is best to make further enquiries to your local council or contact the Department for Education and Skills (DfES).

Available grants

- NHS bursaries
- Dependant's grant
- Childcare grant
- Travel, books and equipment grant
- School meals' grant
- Lone parents' grant
- Disabled students' allowance

14.5 Other financial help available

There are other sources of funds available during term time. These are available to students having financial difficulty. It is necessary to have applied for a full student loan prior to obtaining further support.

Hardship funds

Each university has a pot of money allocated to it by the Government that is to be distributed to those students with financial difficulties. A student loan must have been taken out and other pathways explored before applying for this fund. The amount received will depend on individual circumstances and also the number of students applying. This money does not need to be repaid.

Hardship loan

This is another loan that can be applied for if the full student loan has already been granted. The extra money is normally in the region of £500. This money will be added to your original loan account and needs repaying.

Access to Learning Fund

These funds are to help students encountering particular hardship because of a disability, living costs or childcare. The aim of the fund is to support vulnerable students, in particular to help them access and remain in higher education, for example students who meet unexpected financial crisis or who may be considering leaving their course because of financial problems. Access Fund grants cannot be made for paying tuition fees.

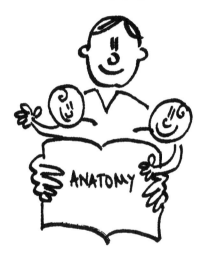

Access funds are now available for students who are parents

Scholarships and awards

These are another way of funding students through university. Most institutions offer them to cover either the whole cost of the course or a contribution to it. There will be differences between the individual universities so, if you feel that extra financial help will be necessary, contact the student support centres.

14.6 Bank loans

Once the above sources of income have been used but money is still necessary to put food on the table, it may be time to look towards a friendly bank manager. On arrival at university you should either convert your current bank account or open a new student account. A better idea would be to open a student account before arrival in your new town; during freshers' week there can be long queues at the banks. Most of the high street banks offer special introductory deals as a temptation. Study these deals carefully because although £50 up front is a good incentive, a better interest rate on an overdraft might save you more money in the long run. There may be better deals around on the internet but having a personal account manager at a local bank can be useful during times of trouble. Discuss the details with the individual banks to decide on which will fit your criteria the best. Most medical schools have cash machines in close proximity. Try to arrange an account manager early on.

It is fair to say that banks are especially sympathetic towards medical students. For this reason it is often possible to arrange larger overdrafts and loans than other students. This is because of the unique situation that a medical student is virtually guaranteed a job following graduation. Remember that the interest rates are not as competitive as student loans.

14.7 Pay back

As a medical student it is possible to borrow a large amount of money during university. Do not forget that this money has to be repaid at some point. The SLC commences repayment in the April of the year following graduation. Anyone earning less than £15 000 does not need to start repayments but this will not be relevant when you are a doctor. Bank loans will be considered on an individual basis but as the interest charges will be much higher, it is best to pay these off as quickly as possible.

14.8 Student employment

One method of preventing such a huge debt at university is to work. Many students take up holiday jobs but this becomes difficult after the third year for medical students. The other option is to actually find part-time employment in your university town. Again this can be more difficult as a medical student because of the rigours of the course, but certainly still possible. Most students opt for evening bar work or Saturday jobs.

14.9 Finance for graduate courses

It is important to mention that graduates gaining admission to the standard 5-year course will be eligible to apply for student loans for their maintenance. If they have previously taken a publicly funded higher education course lasting 2 years or more, they will not be entitled to receive funding from their local authorities for tuition fees and universities may charge them the full cost of their tuition. (Fees payable to medical schools by graduate students vary widely and details are available from the schools themselves.) From year

5 onwards, tuition fees will be paid by the Department of Health and they will be eligible to apply for a means-tested NHS bursary, and reduced maintenance loan from the SLC (equivalent to approximately half the full rate).

Graduates on accelerated (4-year) courses are eligible to apply for means-tested NHS bursaries from the Department of Health in the second, third and fourth years of the course. Tuition fees are also paid during that period of the course. In their first year, graduate students on accelerated courses will be eligible to apply for student loans from the SLC for their maintenance. Information about NHS student bursaries is available at www.nhsbsa.nhs.uk/students.

14.10 Post graduation

In general doctors do not tend to be the most financially astute individuals. This can be a problem if financial priorities are not realized at an early stage. As a newly qualified doctor you will be earning a significant amount of money and there is a temptation to go out and buy extravagant items. The first priority should be to pay off loans.

It is sensible to find a reliable financial adviser at this time. Be cautious in your decision because history has proven that these experts have not always been correct or indeed acted in the best interests of the individual. There are many reputable companies around and recommendation by a colleague is reassuring. Financial advisers can be independent or affiliated to one particular company. The latter can only recommend products by that one company, which can be quite limiting. The other point to check is whether you have to pay for financial advice given or if they obtain commission from the companies directly, following a policy being taken.

Financial advisers can help with advice regarding repayment of debts, pensions, saving for the future, mortgages and income protection. Income protection should be considered following graduation. Once a policy is taken out, your wage will continue to be paid if you need to have a prolonged time off work. Monthly payments are in the region of £30. Following graduation there are other compulsory payments that need to be made annually, including membership of the General Medical Council and indemnity insurance with either the Medical Defence Union or the Medical Protection Society.

Post-graduation outgoings

- General Medical Council
- British Medical Association
- Medical Defence Society
- Income protection
- Postgraduate exams and courses
- Membership of postgraduate college

Wage deductions

- NHS pension contribution
- National Insurance
- Car parking
- Accommodation

Once you are qualified you may have to complete a tax return. It is not within the remit of this book to discuss this in great detail but the following are some helpful hints.

- Any income on top of your normal wage may not have been taxed at source. This includes money obtained from the completion of cremation forms.
- It is necessary to declare this extra income in order to pay the tax.
- It is wise to keep all financial documents, for example bank statements, in a safe place.
- It is possible to complete a tax return personally, but many doctors employ an accountant to do this on their behalf.

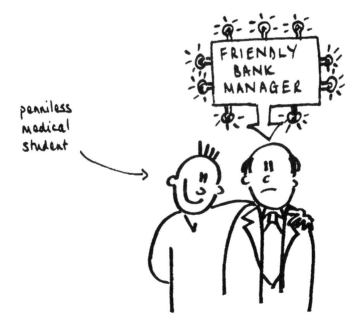

Once sources of income have been drained . . . it may be time to look towards a friendly bank manager

14.11 Summary

University can be expensive, but no student should be deterred from going for financial reasons. There are several available sources of finance for those struggling. The best advice is to budget carefully from the start of the term. Have an income and expenditure spreadsheet and decide how much can be spent on socializing each week. There are certain essential items, for example accommodation and food. Other items will have to be foregone if money is tight, for example mobile phone and alcohol. Each university will be different so contact the student support groups if you think you may be in financial trouble. The earlier this is done the better, because there can be delays in the processing of forms. We cannot recommend getting into debt up to your eyeballs, but do bear in mind that, once qualified, doctors are virtually guaranteed a job and do earn a reasonable income.

Chapter 15 **House dog to top dog**

On completion of medical school, a student has reached the top of a ladder, only to then start at the base of the next one. It will take a doctor several years of training, progressing through the ranks, to become an independent practitioner. This is irrespective of your final career choice, although the length of training will depend on the specialty chosen. This chapter describes the generic career pathway following medical school. The majority of doctors train in the broad areas of surgery, medicine or general practice and a chapter has been dedicated to each of these areas (see Chapters 19, 20 and 21).

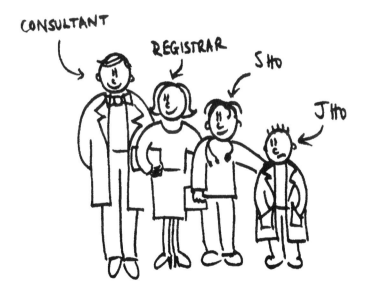

Teams of doctors in hospitals are referred to as firms

The Essential Guide to Becoming a Doctor, 3rd edition. © Adrian Blundell, Richard Harrison and Benjamin Turney. Published 2011 by Blackwell Publishing Ltd.

Since the first edition of this book in 2001, the postgraduate medical training structure has undergone major reform. Many of the changes are still in their infancy and there will no doubt be continued tweaking over the next few years. For a historical prospective we will discuss the old system first and then describe the new structure. The changes have been overseen by the Modernizing Medical Careers (MMC) group and for the most up-to-date information we recommend reviewing their website (www.mmc.nhs.uk).

Further essential information can be found at the British Medical Association (BMA) website. The BMA is the professional association and trade union for doctors in the UK and the website has information for all levels of students and doctors, with important documents updated annually (www.bma.org.uk).

15.1 The old system

Figure 15.1 summarizes the previous postgraduate career ladder. Following successful graduation, a medical student became a pre-registration house

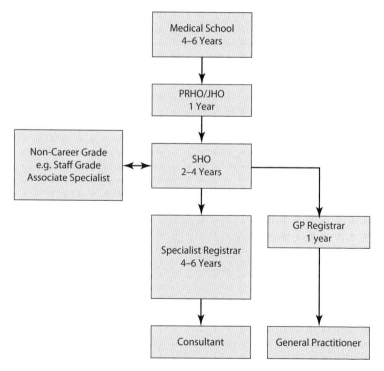

Figure 15.1 Simplified diagrammatic representation of the old training ladder for doctors (see text for details).

officer (PRHO), previously known as a junior house officer (JHO), or more affectionately as House Officer, House Plant or House Dog! Pre-registration basically reflected the fact that newly qualified doctors are automatically granted provisional registration with the General Medical Council (GMC). This post lasted 12 months and usually consisted of two (or occasionally three) rotations at a couple of different hospitals. The rotations were generally divided into 6 months of medical specialty jobs and then 6 months of surgical positions. If successful at completing the first year, a doctor could then fully register with the GMC and apply for the next post, which would be at senior house officer (SHO) level. The SHO jobs could either be stand-alone 6-month positions (e.g. accident and emergency) or a doctor could enter a 2- or 3-year 'rotation' in a chosen field, for example medicine, surgery or paediatrics (see Chapter 18). Many doctors also took the opportunity to work abroad at some point during their early years. Following the completion of a specialty SHO rotation and postgraduate exams, a doctor could then apply to become a specialist registrar (SpR) in a subspecialty area (e.g. cardiology). Doctors training to become general practitioners would complete 2 years as an SHO and 1 year as a GP registrar and would then be eligible to be independent practitioners. SpR training usually lasted between 4 and 6 years and often included further examinations. Once complete, a doctor would be eligible to gain a certificate of completion of specialist training (CCST) and become a consultant.

15.2 Modernizing Medical Careers

Over the last 10 years, attempts have been made to change medical training for the better. The introduction of the PRHO year and the SpR grade following a report in 1993 by the then Chief Medical Officer Kenneth Calman made some improvements. There was still the problem at the SHO level, with wide variety in the quality and consistency of jobs. There was no clear career pathway and continued problems between training and service commitment. MMC was devised to help streamline this training of junior doctors from graduation up to the point of independent practice. The main difference between the systems is that progress through training will no longer be determined by time spent but by evidence of the outcomes of training, demonstrated through competency-based assessment with the overall aim of having focused streamlined training for all grades. In principle this should mean better training, more supervision, increased flexibility and defined competencies to be gained before progression to the next level. The reality is still uncertain but is likely to mean increased paperwork (in the form of more detailed training portfolios), an increase in the number of assessments and probably a less experienced workforce in more senior positions. Another drawback that has been seen since the implementation of MMC is greater competition for jobs, making the profession even more competitive.

15.3 The Foundation Programme

The Foundation Programme is a 2-year programme of general training that was implemented in August 2005 and has been introduced to form a bridge between medical school and specialist/general practice training. Medical students will apply for a Foundation Programme place during their final year. A website dedicated to all aspects of the Foundation Programme can be accessed at www.foundationprogramme.nhs.uk.

Over the 2 years a doctor will rotate through a number of specialties in various healthcare settings. Rather than just experiencing general medicine and surgery, the Foundation Programme will allow a greater choice of attachments (e.g. anaesthetics, general practice, psychiatry). This enables greater variety at an earlier stage, which could help with future career decisions. The placements will each last 4 months, which potentially means some time could be spent in up to eight specialties. Emphasis will still be placed on the importance of medical and surgical specialties, so most programmes will include two medical and surgical jobs. The postgraduate training involved in the Foundation Programme is organized locally by the postgraduate deanery and will be administered through so-called foundation schools. These schools will consist of medical schools, local deaneries and other healthcare providers such as the acute hospitals, primary care trusts and organizations such as hospices. This will enable an increased variety of specialties and also settings in which to work (e.g. acute hospitals, community, mental health and general practice). There are 26 foundation schools as of 2010, with each being responsible for around 300 doctors. There is a plan for several of these to merge in the near future.

With the introduction of this new programme, there has also been a change in the format of application for jobs. Previously each university was affiliated with enough PRHO placements for the number of graduates. The majority of the posts were located in the same geographic region and each student applied through a local computer-matching scheme with their preferences. The application system completely changed in 2007 with a national online service called the Medical Training Application Service (MTAS). Unfortunately, there were multiple problems with this system and it was scrapped, leaving a great number of disgruntled doctors and also considerable embarrassment for the Government. The fiasco resulted in a new lobbying group being formed by a collection of junior doctors to challenge changes in training and employment strategies (see www.remedyuk.org for more information).

Since 2008, medical students apply for a Foundation Programme placement using the online application process available at www.foundationprogramme. nhs.uk. The application process involves the completion of an online form. Following the application, an overall score is given to each candidate comprising an academic score provided by their medical school and a score relating to their application answers. The closing date for applications is towards the end of October in the final year. As part of the application, students need to rank the foundation schools in order of preference. If candidates do not get their first-choice foundation school, their documentation is automatically forwarded to their next ranked choice of school. This process may be repeated until all available places are filled. Students will then be matched to a 2-year Foundation Programme, attracting a 2-year contract of employment.

The first year of the Foundation Programme (Foundation Year 1, FY1 or F1), is similar to the old PRHO year, building on the knowledge, skills and competencies acquired during university. Instead of two 6-month placements, this year will be divided into 4-month attachments. The GMC, along with the local postgraduate deanery, are currently responsible for this stage of training and F1 trainees will need to demonstrate areas of competence outlined in the GMC's booklet *The New Doctor* in order to be recommended for full registration at the end of the first year.

The first Foundation Year 2 (FY2 or F2) programmes began in August 2006. The F2 year equates to the previous SHO year 1 but the jobs will consist of three 4-month placements. The Postgraduate Medical Education and Training Board (PMETB), along with the deanery, currently have responsibility for postgraduate training from this year onwards. The emphasis during this second year is again on achieving core competencies as outlined in the joint MMC/Academy of Medical Royal Colleges curriculum. This will build on the skills developed during the first year and also concentrate on other more generic issues such as team-working, communication skills and use of evidence-based medicine.

The foundation programmes should, within a structured programme, deliver training in the broad generic competencies that every doctor will need during his or her career. They are designed to give trainees the opportunity to experience a range of clinical settings. Both F1 and F2 trainees will need to provide evidence that the competencies outlined in the curriculum have been achieved and this will be helped by developing a training portfolio and using newly introduced assessment tools where doctors' skills are directly observed. Each doctor is allocated an educational supervisor who will be a senior clinician, not directly working with the trainee. The supervisor will organize regular meetings to review the progress and run through an appraisal process. The training portfolio will be used at these meetings to check the doctor is progressing appropriately. Each doctor also has his or her own consultant to assist in progression and during the year will have a couple of review meetings with the foundation programme director (another senior consultant). This director is responsible for signing trainees off, to enable them to progress to the next stage of training. If adequate competencies have not been achieved, then a doctor may need to repeat all or some of the year. In principle these changes would seem to be for the better, but the reality is currently unclear – spending less time in more jobs could actually equate to doctors being less experienced at the basics.

Advantages of the Foundation Programme

- Trainee centred
- Single UK curriculum defining training over the 2 years
- Nationally agreed training portfolio
- Named educational supervisor
- Regular reviews and appraisals
- Increased variety of placements
- Competency-based assessments
- Single application process
- Increased supervision initially

Disadvantages of the Foundation Programme

- National application process
- More paperwork and ticking boxes
- Less time in each post
- More supernumerary positions
- Less experienced at the end due to shorter hours
- Too much supervision

15.4 Specialty training

Once the Foundation Programme is complete, the majority of doctors will commence specialty training (job title: specialty registrar), which lasts between 5 and 8 years depending on the chosen specialty. Applications for specialty training (hospital or community) take place during the F2 year.

This means that doctors need to decide relatively early in their career as to what specialty they wish to pursue. There are a range of specialties to choose from, some of which offer 'run-through' training, i.e. once on the next rung of the ladder a trainee is guaranteed promotion until completion of training, while others offer generic training for the first 2 or 3 years prior to a doctor having to apply for a further training post in a subspecialty area for their final 4–5 years. The box below summarizes the choice of parent specialties available in 2010. The application procedure still involves a centralized online application but instead of MTAS it is organized by a royal college or a nominated deanery. The process varies slightly for each specialty and more information, including indicative competition ratios, is available in Chapters 18–21 and also at www.mmc.nhs.uk.

Specialties offering run-through training at specialty registrar grade

- Chemical pathology
- Clinical radiology
- General practice
- Histopathology
- Medical microbiology/virology
- Neurosurgery
- Obstetrics and gynaecology
- Ophthalmology
- Paediatrics and child health
- Public health medicine
- Trauma and orthopaedic surgery

Specialties offering uncoupled training at specialty registrar grade

- Anaesthetics
- Core medical training (for medical specialties not listed elsewhere)
- Core surgical training (for surgical specialties not listed elsewhere)
- Emergency medicine
- Psychiatry

The specialty training years involve a new integrated streamlined training that combines the previous SHO and SpR grades. The main reason for this change was the lack of structure to the SHO grade. The aim now is to have a well-organized and structured programme with a clear curriculum within a seamless training process incorporating both the grades. Progress throughout the programme will be through competency-based assessment (in a similar way

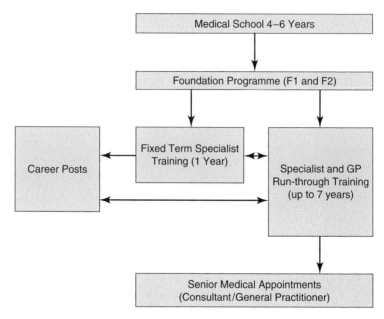

Figure 15.2 Simplified diagrammatic representation of the proposed generic training ladder for doctors (see text for details).

to the Foundation Programme). The curricula are overseen by the PMETB and the medical royal colleges. The training programmes will initially be broad-based, with increased specialization as a trainee progresses. After completion of a specialty training programme, a doctor will gain a certificate of completion, be legally eligible for entry to the specialist or GP register and can then apply for an appropriate senior medical appointment. Figure 15.2 summarizes the MMC framework.

15.5 Fixed-term specialist training and career posts

Not all doctors will be successful at obtaining a specialty training post and some may choose to delay for a while. Fixed-term specialist training posts are 1-year appointments in a given specialty. The training will be the same as for a trainee in the run-through programme without the natural progression. The options after completing the year are to apply for an appropriate specialist training post and hence get back on the training ladder, or apply for a non-consultant career grade post in an appropriate specialty. The non-consultant career grade posts are service delivery positions, meaning there is no formalized specialty training elements. The posts are only available in secondary care and a doctor will need to have completed at least 3 years of post-registration training before taking on such an appointment. Figure 15.2 shows in more detail where these posts fit in to the MMC framework. The posts used to carry titles such as staff grade doctor or associate specialist but since 2008 a new title of specialty doctor has been introduced. These are positions that can be taken if a doctor does not wish to become a consultant or is unable to do so for either educational or personal reasons. Several years experience in the hospital specialty is necessary, but these posts do not require a doctor to be on the specialist register and for this reason they are responsible to a named consultant and hence not completely independent practitioners.

15.6 Advantages and disadvantages of the specialty training programme

Advantages
- Seamless progression from foundation programmes to specialist training.
- Broadly based specialty training at first, progressing to greater specialization.
- Flexibility if career aspirations change, with recognition of previous experience.
- Rigorous in-training assessment.
- Flexibility to allow the pursuit of academia, out-of-programme experience and the opportunity to train less than full-time.
- Good career counselling and efficient manpower planning.

Disadvantages
- Less specialist training places.
- May produce less experienced consultants.
- National centralized online application process leading to less personalization.
- The possible introduction of a new sub-consultant grade.
- More difficult to work abroad.
- Earlier decision needed over which specialty to pursue.

15.7 Senior medical appointments

Once specialty training has been completed, a Certificate of Completion of Training (CCT) is awarded, and a doctor is then eligible to apply for a senior medical appointment. These positions include GP principals, consultants and other employed GPs. This means that a doctor is qualified to practice independently and with that has the ultimate responsibility for the patients under his or her care (the Top Dog!). Once doctors have reached the level of consultant, they may also carry out private work in addition to their NHS commitments.

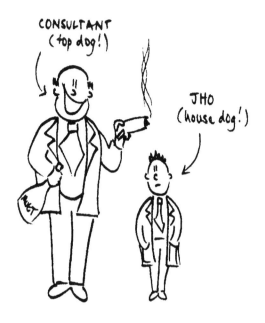

15.8 Summary

There have been major changes in the postgraduate training structure for doctors over the last 5 years. This chapter has introduced the generic training structure for doctors regardless of specialty. The nomenclature can be confusing and the table below describes the titles used in the medical profession. Figure 15.2 shows the generic training structure and where the different grades fit into this. Postgraduate training is obviously far in the future for any premedical school student, but it is certainly worth keeping abreast of any changes by reviewing the websites suggested in this chapter; it is certainly a topic that could be asked at interview. The other concern is that the training structures are still in their infancy and are being scrutinized closely. The Foundation Programme structure is being reviewed during 2010 to verify that it is fit for purpose – it may be the case that it is eventually uncoupled, reverting to a system similar to that of the past!

Medical Student	Medical students will spend 4–6 years training to become a doctor
Foundation Year 1 Doctor (FY1)	Following successful graduation, a student will become an FY1 doctor. These posts used to be termed Junior House Officer (JHO) or Pre-Registration House Officer (PRHO)
Foundation Year 2 Doctor (FY2)	If the FY1 year is completed satisfactorily, most doctors will automatically become FY2 doctors. This grade was previously known as Senior House Officer (SHO)
Specialty Registrar (ST1–ST7)	FY2 doctors can apply for specialty training in one of the parent specialties shown in section 15.4. Competition for places increases as a doctor climbs the training ladder. These posts are the equivalent of the old SHO and SpR grades. Doctors are known as Specialty Training Registrars
Consultant	Following completion of specialty training and postgraduate examinations, a doctor may apply to become a consultant
General Practitioner	Following completion of GP specialty training and a postgraduate qualification, a doctor may apply to become a principal GP or a salaried GP. A principal GP is a partner of a practice whereas a salaried GP is employed by a practice
Specialty Doctor	If for training or personal reasons a doctor decides not to complete training to become a GP or consultant, then it is possible to take up a post in a non-consultant career grade. These doctors used to be termed staff grade or associate specialists
Professor	This title is conferred on those who reach the highest level in the medical profession who have followed an academic pathway (see Chapter 18). Doctors who follow such a path have slightly different titles during their training, such as lecturer, senior lecturer, reader and associate professor

PERSONAL VIEW (2006)   *Bryony Elliott*

I am writing this vignette as a pre-registration house officer (PRHO) 6 months after graduation from the University of Nottingham Medical School. I am one of many doctors in the first 'guinea-pig' year of the Foundation Programme. As with every new system there have been surprising developments along the

(continued)

(*Continued*)

way. During the application process there did not seem to be a long-term itinerary for when things would happen, or indeed how. It all seemed to be a case of trial and error. Thankfully, the Trent deanery pushed the boat out and organized 2-year rotations where other deaneries throughout the country were only organizing FY1 posts. This allowed me and many of my peers to plan the next 2 years of our lives. The process started with a complicated online application form. We had to give evidence of situations in which we had shown particular characteristics, list fourth-year examination grades and provide details of two referees. Along with this we had to rank our choice of jobs. Individuals had to decide where they wanted to work and which jobs incorporated the specialties they wanted to experience. We were then ranked, based on our application forms and matched to our choice of jobs, by what felt like a completely random process. The majority of my friends did well. The deanery reported that about 70% of my year got one of their top three jobs. However, I had friends who for no apparent reason did not get matched and had to go through an extra clearing stage. It never became clear why they were so unlucky, and they certainly never got feedback on which part of the application had let them down.

Happily I got my first-ranked job and am currently on a 2-year rotation that will include general medicine, urology, general practice, cardiology, obstetrics and gynaecology, and trauma and orthopaedics. I consider myself lucky that I will be able to experience all these specialties before choosing which path I want to take, because like a lot of people I still don't have a clue where I want to end up! This seems much more satisfying than the old system during which I would have done 6 months of medicine and 6 months of surgery, and then had to decide on my career path. On the flip side, however, there are some people in my year who are certain about their career path. They feel that they are just passing time in different specialties waiting to apply for the specialty training programme of their choice. Similarly, there is a question whether people who have had experience of a specialty in their Foundation Programme will be looked upon more favourably in the application process for specialty training. This seems a little unfair on people who did not get a Foundation Programme with a particular specialty or for those who have had a change of heart on the career front.

My day-to-day job is much like it would have been in the old system, and in my view a vital part of the development of any junior doctor. I provide a service, which is like being the ward dogsbody. It certainly lacks the glamour of *ER*! I take blood, chase the results, and make sure the results of scans and tests are in the notes ready for more senior review. However, it is in my power to make a big difference to patient care. With no clinic or theatre commitments it is the FY1 trainees who have the time to talk to patients and their families. At the heart of it, the FY1 trainee is on the ground as the first port of call, dealing with patients. If the nurses are worried about someone they call the junior doctor, and it is this exposure to acutely unwell patients that improves your clinical and diagnostic skills.

As a Foundation Programme trainee I have been allocated an educational supervisor (someone independent to my working team) to help me keep track of my long-term aims and progress, and a clinical supervisor (my consultant) who gives feedback on my working practice. There are timetabled meetings throughout the year at which we have to document our discussions and plan further appointments. In my opinion this has been valuable and a welcome development in junior doctor training. I feel like I have a structured support network of people who I can turn to for support and, perhaps more importantly, advice about where my career is going from here.

As part of the training I have to keep a portfolio, much like the RITA (Record of In Training Assessment) kept by more senior doctors. This is evidence of procedures I have carried out and experience I have gained. There are set aims and objectives that all training schemes nationwide have to adhere to. In reality this means I have protected 1-hour teaching sessions once a week, during which the Trust supplies teaching on core topics in the curriculum. The theory is that by the end of both the FY1 and the FY2 years, each and every doctor will have completed the core competencies before moving on to further training. These competencies are tested by a variety of assessments, from peer review tools to direct observation in a clinical setting. Trainees are also encouraged to actively reflect on their practice and how they have dealt with certain situations. The idea is that doctors are being encouraged to recognize their strengths and weaknesses and identify areas for improvement.

I have really enjoyed working life so far. As a student I used to feel that I got in the way and it is great to finally have a role. I do sometimes feel like a small cog in a very large machine, and it is easy to think that the mundane administrative tasks are unimportant. But then I remind myself that if I did not fill in the form and take it to the radiologist, my patient would not get the necessary scan, and the diagnosis would be delayed. Working for the NHS involves being part of a massive team. I have met hundreds of people since I

(continued)

(*Continued*)

have started working and the people I work with have been a big part of my life. The majority of the FY1 trainees live in hospital accommodation and there is a great camaraderie and an active social life. I am excited by the chance to experience a diverse range of specialties in the next 2 years, and hopefully somewhere along the line I will come up with a plan for the future.

PERSONAL VIEW (2010)   *Bryony Elliott*

It is interesting to reflect on my progression since writing my first vignette nearly 4 years ago. As then, throughout my training I have been on the frontier of changes in medical training. I completed the Foundation Programme and jumped through the hoops of MMC, only to abruptly collide with the wall of MTAS. I survived that hurdle and am now a Specialty Registrar (ST3) in geriatric medicine, on the final straight to consultantdom.

The theory was that every trainee finishing the Foundation Programme throughout the country would apply for specialty training posts through a centralized application process. We were given four job choices, combining specialty and area. By this point I knew that I wanted to pursue a career in a medical specialty. I had loved my geriatric and cardiology jobs in the Foundation Programme and successfully ruled out obstetrics and gynaecology, which had been my main contender on leaving medical school.

Halfway through our FY2 year we started the process of applying for 'run-through' (ST1–ST7) training, the golden ticket of guaranteed training to consultant level. This was a new concept: job security in one place for the remainder of your training. I knew that I wanted to stay in the Trent region, if I stayed in the UK at all. I had bought a flat and felt settled here. My theory was that I would apply for core medical training in Trent, using only one of my possible four choices, and if I did not get the job I would emigrate to Australia – it was in the hands of fate!

Along with the rest of the trainees at my level in that year, I filled in the online application form. Different specialties had slightly different questions on their forms, but essentially if you were applying for one specialty in four regions then you had one online form to complete. The process was fairly simple for me because I had applied to one region (I got an interview and subsequently got a job offer), but I watched as my friends received their job offers and considered which they would accept before the final deadline. Some people were lucky and got the specialty of their choice in the area they wanted to live. Others had to decide between FTSTA offers in the area they wanted, or a 'run-through' job in a less favourable region.

MTAS was considered a disaster; the press had a field day. The logistics of filling posts neatly and mathematically did not compute with real life. Good doctors struggled to get jobs, especially those caught in the last couple of years of SHO jobs that were too qualified for the new ST1/2 posts. Deaneries have tried several recruitment methods over the last few years and have now ironed out some of the kinks. Medicine has opted again for a nationalized process coordinated by the Royal College of Physicians. They have also realized that the realities of life mean that not all candidates are suitable for higher training and the 'run-through' training system has been decoupled, moving back to a system much like the old one, where ST1 and ST2 are considered core medical training and ST3 upwards as higher specialist training. However, they had to honour our appointments and in our year we had an internal competitive entry process for subspecialty training at ST3.

I've now climbed the ranks. My role has changed from being a ward monkey to being a senior member of the team, involved in more complicated management decisions. I do clinics, sessions at the community hospital and have time for professional development, in addition to my ward work. The focus is on my training and the skills I need to acquire before I can be an independent practitioner. The system of educational and clinical supervisor support has continued throughout my training and has provided a structured record of my career progression. The workplace-based assessments (WPBA) have remained and I have moved through the paper-based NHS portfolio onto the newer e-portfolio, an online logbook recording my training. Although time-consuming to keep up to date, WPBAs have become an integral part of modern practice and gradually more and more seniors are engaging appropriately with the system.

Things have changed extensively in the last 4 years. FY1 doctors no longer have hospital accommodation provided. Working hours have been cut in line with the European Working Time Directive and consequently juniors are on basic salaries with no additional pay. This has an impact on repaying student loans and could be a factor in deciding on medicine as a career. I am glad that I trained when I have. Although I have had to work within new systems, I think they have been implemented for the better. I have benefited from some great initiatives and luckily managed to avoid the pitfalls along the way. Now I just have to concentrate on working towards that position as Top Dog!

Chapter 16 **Working patterns and wages**

16.1 Recent changes

Before discussing the various working patterns and pay schemes for junior doctors, it is necessary to mention some of the changes seen within the health service over the last few years. Until fairly recently it was not uncommon for a junior doctor to be working over 100 hours in a single week. Research has shown that tired doctors do not function to the best of their abilities. There can be an effect on a doctor's performance, which can lead to safety issues for the patients, but there can also be direct effects on the health and well-being of the individual doctor. This can then escalate and lead to problems with social and family life. By the 1990s these potential problems had been realized, and it was decided that regulations should be imposed on the maximum number of hours that doctors should be working in a week. The reduction in hours also meant that there needed to be a change in working patterns. More information and up-to-date guidance on hours and wages can be found on the BMA website (www.bma.org.uk/) and by reading the BMA's *Junior Doctors' Handbook*.

16.2 The New Deal

Because of the great concern about the long hours that junior doctors were working, the Government, NHS personnel and doctor representatives agreed, in 1991, on a new working practice for training doctors. This was called *Junior Doctors: The New Deal*. As well as trying to reduce the number of hours, this document also aimed to improve such issues as doctors' accommodation and provision of food within the hospital out of hours. Until this time, shift work was rare and the majority of doctors were

The Essential Guide to Becoming a Doctor, 3rd edition. © Adrian Blundell,
Richard Harrison and Benjamin Turney. Published 2011 by Blackwell Publishing Ltd.

working on-call rosters. The New Deal suggested that the introduction of shift patterns could help reduce the number of hours worked (the types of rota are discussed in the next section). By the end of 1996, the maximum number of hours worked per week for each different type of shift had been decided: 72 hours for on-call, 64 hours for partial shift, and 56 hours for full shift. As well as this, it was decided that the average working week over the full contract of the job should average no more than 56 hours per week.

The New Deal hours implementation

1994	No doctor should be working more than 56 hours (on average) per week
1996	Maximum hours per week for the different shifts implemented (e.g. 72 hours for on-call)
2000	Actual *contractual* requirement for limits on hours
2001	*All* New Deal hour limits and rest requirements contractual for PRHO grade
2003	As 2001 but for *all* other training doctors

Unfortunately, although the Government advised this legislation, hospitals in general were extremely slow to implement any changes. Even by 2002 almost one-third of junior doctors were still working outside the New Deal limits. To improve this situation, further measures were taken in 2000 as part of the new Junior Doctor Contract, which was negotiated by the Junior Doctors Committee (JDC). This stated that the New Deal hours per week and rest requirements would become a contractual obligation for a hospital when new doctors were employed. This meant that in essence it would be illegal for a hospital to employ a doctor on a contract that was outside the New Deal guidelines. The deadline for PRHO posts was August 2001 and for other training doctors August 2003. To determine the actual number of hours worked in a week, it is necessary for the junior doctors to monitor their hours – this is also a contractual obligation. If they are found to be outside the New Deal target, hospital trusts are at risk of losing recognition for the posts (i.e. they risk losing the doctors).

16.3 Junior doctor working patterns

There are different types of rota currently used by hospitals for junior doctors. This will not only depend on which hospital you work at but also the specialty you have chosen.

On-call

Historically, most training doctors, regardless of specialty, worked this rota. For this pattern, a doctor would work a normal day (9 a.m. to 5 p.m.) followed by an on-call period from 5 p.m. until 9 a.m. the next morning and then another normal 9 to 5 day (a total of 32 hours). During the on-call period, it would be expected that a doctor would be working for only half this time, the rest of the time being spent resting, preferably with some sleep (i.e. at least 8 hours rest); in reality, on-call for many jobs is actually busier than the normal working day. This rota could also include working at the weekend: a doctor would work Saturday morning until Monday evening (a total of 56 hours). On-call rotas are now rare; they are mainly used for senior doctors and those junior doctors working in non-acute specialties (e.g. public health medicine).

Partial shift

These rotas became more common towards the late 1990s. Doctors work a combination of shifts to cover the emergency work but the majority of their time should be spent within working hours, i.e. 9 a.m. to 5 p.m. The maximum shift length allowed was 16 hours but 4 hours compulsory rest was required. With this shift pattern doctors will take it in turns to work night shifts and, when working at night, have the following day to sleep.

Full shift

These shifts are commonly used in other professions. In medicine the most common specialty to use a full shift pattern is A&E (accident and emergency). The whole rota is of a shift variety, with no routine 9 to 5 days. The maximum time allowed to work each shift is 14 hours, although most shifts will be between 8 and 12 hours.

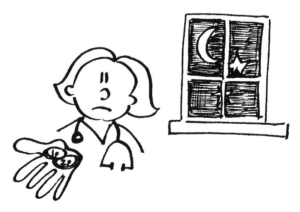

. . . which meant that a doctor would earn a third of her normal wage when working on call

Hybrid rota

This is a combination of the above. The table below shows the hours of work and rest with each of the different shift patterns. The introduction of the European Working Time Directive (EWTD) has now superseded some of the rules with regard to maximum number of hours and rest periods (see next section).

Working pattern	Maximum continuous period of duty (hours)	Minimum period off between duties (hours)	Minimum rest during the duty
Full shift	14	8	Natural breaks
Partial shift	16	8	¼ out-of-hours duty
On-call	32 (56 at weekend)	12	½ out-of-hours duty

16.4 The European Working Time Directive

This directive is European law and was introduced to protect the health and safety of all workers within the European Union (not just doctors). It was introduced in 1998 but initially junior doctors were not included. After discussions in 2000, it was decided that the new legislation would affect junior doctors and that the changes would be incorporated over the next 9–11 years. The main effects on working hours are summarized below.

European Working Time Directive timetable

August 2004
- 58-hour maximum working week
- Rest and break requirements enforced

August 2007
- 56-hour maximum working week

August 2009
- 48-hour maximum working week
- Possibly extended to 2012 with 52-hour week in 2009

The changes in rest requirements become compulsory in 2004 and are summarized below.

> **European Working Time Directive rest requirements (by 2004)**
>
> - Minimum daily consecutive rest period 11 hours, i.e. maximum shift 13 hours
> - Minimum rest period of 24 hours in each 7-day period or 48 hours in 14 days
> - Minimum rest break of 20 minutes if shift exceeds 6 hours
> - Minimum 4 weeks paid annual leave
> - All hours spent at hospital counted as actual work
> - Maximum of 8 hours work in any 24 hours for night-workers in stressful jobs

As one can see, long hours for junior doctors should not necessarily be a problem now or in the future. It is worth noting though that the hours worked are calculated as an average over a set period and so doctors often work more than 48 hours in a week but then get compensatory rest periods at another time. The advantages and disadvantages are discussed later in this chapter.

16.5 The new pay system

The traditional pay system for junior doctors consisted of a basic salary, which would cover the normal working day, and then an hourly rate for time spent on-call, which was classed as additional duty hours (ADHs). ADHs were divided into categories depending on the intensity of the work out of hours. Most jobs were defined as being class 3, which in real terms meant a doctor would earn a third of his or her normal wage when working on-call. This should have represented the fact that the doctor would only actually be working for a third of the time (i.e. 8 hours rest in a 24-hour period). Unfortunately, as discussed earlier, the intensity of many jobs was such that very little rest was obtained – in summary, a fairly poor deal.

December 2000 saw the end of ADHs and the introduction of a new banding system. The basic salary remains the same but now a doctor will receive a supplemental payment corresponding to the amount of out-of-hours work performed. The supplement is calculated as a proportion of the basic salary and depends on the working pattern, total hours worked and the antisocial nature of a post. Those posts with longer and more antisocial hours are rewarded with a greater supplement.

The new system is divided into four bands (bands 1 and 2 are further subdivided into A and B).

The banding levels

Band 3
- All doctors whose jobs are non-compliant with the New Deal (see above)

Band 2
- Jobs compliant with the New Deal and working over 48 hours but less than 56 hours per week

Band 1
- Jobs compliant with the New Deal and working less than 48 hours per week

Band F
- Jobs over 40 hours per week

Financially, it is obviously much better to be working a job with a band 3 wage but socially not so! Unfortunately, these jobs are not compliant with the New Deal or EWTD and so are in essence illegal. There have been virtually no jobs paid at band 3 since 2005 and with the current financial climate most hospitals have now devised compliant rotas, so most doctors are on band 1. It is recommended to keep abreast of developments and if you are interested in finding out more, look at the BMA website.

16.6 Is change for the better?

Are there only advantages to reducing the number of hours that a junior doctor works? From the surface it would seem that fewer hours is a great idea. Certainly patient safety is of paramount importance and it has been shown that a tired doctor could risk making more mistakes. As well as patient safety, other advantages include the positive effect working fewer hours should have on the health and well-being of a doctor. This in turn should lead to better enjoyment of family and social life.

It is important to look at the argument from both sides and consider this matter even at an early stage as it can be asked at interview. The box below summarizes some of the disadvantages to shift working. One disadvantage is the loss of the traditional 'firm' structure for teams of doctors. Consequently, there will be disruption to the continuity of care of patients and the disadvantages that this may bring. Already we are seeing patients who change wards while they are in hospital and sometimes see a different doctor each day – not good for the patient or the doctor. Another concern

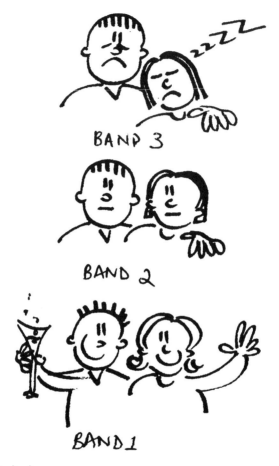

The banding levels

is that a reduction in hours could lead to reduced exposure and experience. Leaders in the surgical specialties are particularly worried about this aspect; for surgery a patient needs a doctor who has spent the relevant time cutting in the operating theatre. One argument against this is that other countries (e.g. in Europe and Australia) have much shorter training programmes with no ill effect on the quality of the doctors produced. It is also felt that if a doctor is less tired, then it is possible to get quality training in a shorter period of time. One other disadvantage is that although the total number of hours will be reduced, full shift rotas often mean an increase in the amount of antisocial hours worked.

Disadvantages to shift working

- Loss of patient continuity
- Working more weekends
- Reduced exposure to clinical conditions
- Possible training opportunities missed
- Fewer hours in the week for learning skills
- Loss of the hospital firm structure of doctors

The current reality is that doctors often find themselves working in different teams each time they are at work and patients are often unsure who their actual doctors are – neither satisfactory. With the reduction in hours, the experience of junior doctors is also being reduced, which can lead to increased pressure on the more senior doctors, and with the government wanting to lower the total number of years of training we may end up with less experienced senior doctors running the show. The best advice is to research thoroughly the jobs you are applying for and check through the contracts carefully before signing them.

16.7 Flexible training in hospital

Another recent improvement has been the awareness of an increased need for flexible training. This enables doctors to work less than full-time but still in posts that are recognized and count towards training. Traditionally, this has been useful for those doctors with family commitments and in general the opportunities have been taken up by many mothers (see Personal view by Anna Rich at the end of this chapter). More recently, individuals with other reasons have decided to train flexibly (see Personal view by Tim Brabants) and consideration will be taken if a doctor has 'well-founded individual reasons'. These can include sporting commitments, family life and problems with ill health. The possibility of flexible training and the number of flexible years allowed depends on the specialty; some of the training time may need to be full-time. An applicant needs to discuss the possibility of flexible training with the relevant postgraduate deanery. There are three options for flexible training: slot share, job share and supernumerary. Slot share is where two doctors share a post, working approximately 60% each so there is overlap, which is useful for continuity. Job share posts are not encouraged and literally mean that two doctors work 50% each of one post. Supernumerary posts are when a doctor is training in addition to the number of required trainees and there is a lack of another suitable flexible trainee and so slot share is not possible.

Doctors who take up GP positions often find flexible training easier and this is certainly the case as a salaried GP (see Chapter 19 for more information).

16.8 The loot

So 5 years at university and up to £20 000 of debt – is it all worth it and, more to the point, how long until that Porsche purchase? Doctors earn a comfortable salary but few will become mega-earners. Financial gain is certainly not a reason for becoming a doctor, especially as it could take several years to pay off all the debts. Newly qualified doctors in particular have noticed a reduction in their wages, especially for those with supernumerary or low banded jobs. In addition, since the dramatic reduction in hours, the free accommodation that used to be provided for FY1 doctors has been revoked and so the cost of living has increased. Some GPs can earn in excess of hospital consultants, but private practice in certain specialties can be lucrative (e.g. surgery). In general the wages reflect responsibility and hence there is an increase as a doctor becomes more senior. The table below summarizes some of the pay scales. These are the basic salaries and do not incorporate the banding supplements. The banding supplements can be calculated as follows: band 1C, 20%; band 1B, 40%; bands 1A and 2B, 50%; band 2A, 80%; and band 3, 100% (e.g. if a doctor was earning £20 000 basic in a band 3 post, the actual wage would be £40 000). Consultants' wages are more complicated and generally higher than the table suggests because over time they earn additional supplements, for example clinical excellence, discretionary points and distinction awards. The final salary of a partnered GP will depend on the income of the whole practice.

Grade	Minimum wage (£)	Maximum wage (£)
FY1	22 190	24 960
FY2	27 523	31 122
Specialty registrar	29 411	46 246
Consultant	74 504	100 446

16.9 Summary

The introduction of the New Deal and the EWTD have seen a reduction in the number of hours that junior doctors work. It is important to be aware of this prior to your application because these are topics that could be discussed at interview. Try to appreciate that there are both advantages and disadvantages to the changes. Potential medical students often ask about doctors' salaries and can be surprised how little a newly qualified doctor earns. While most doctors will not become mega-rich, the salary certainly allows a comfortable life.

PERSONAL VIEW   *Anna Rich*

Opportunities to train flexibly do vary between medical specialties and it may be that this contributes to the career path you choose. I went through medical school assuming I would become a GP, because I knew I wanted a family and knew that you could train and work part-time as a GP. But when I finished my 6 months as a medical House Officer (long before MMC and CMT was invented!). I knew I had found a job I could enjoy long term. I loved being part of the medical firm and my learned consultant advised me that I should choose the career I actually wanted to do, rather than the one I had assumed I would do. I can clearly remember him saying that he felt sure there would be opportunities to train flexibly within hospital medicine before too long, and he was right.

There are lots of different reasons for wanting to train flexibly – combining medicine with sporting brilliance, or health reasons – but for the majority it is so that we can combine medicine with raising our children. Experiences will differ, and I can only describe my own, as a mother of two and a final year Respiratory SpR. One thing to accept from the outset is that you will watch doctors younger than you pass through the training system at 'full-time' speed and complete their training before you. This can be frustrating, but hey, I've not worked a Friday (except the odd on-call) since 2003 and that has definitely been good for my work/life balance.

I must say that I think flexible training would be almost impossible without both supportive senior and registrar colleagues. I have been privileged to have supportive consultants at every NHS Trust that I've worked in since my first pregnancy, and am now doing research as part of an MD part-time (80% FTE). My position has been more appealing to the Trust as I have been funded as a supernumerary trainee and so in effect I am an extra pair of hands. However, this does not mean that I have been idle. Often my presence has allowed one of the full-time trainees to take some time off to write up their research, do an 'out-of-programme experience' (OOPE) slot, or simply to get to some radiology teaching that they usually have to miss out on. Until I started my MD 18 months ago, I worked at 70% FTE, i.e. 3.5 days. This comprised 3 days in hospital and a half day a week of private study leave. In those 3 days I would be timetabled for my own and one consultant ward round, I would have a bronchoscopy list, and then usually two clinics, leaving a half day for referrals. This is a comparable timetable to my full-time colleagues, who would have perhaps one extra consultant ward round a week. The result is that my senior and registrar colleagues appreciate that while I'm not there all the time,

(continued)

(*Continued*)

when I am there I'm working hard. And I have honestly found that I do not get involved with any ward 'politics' nor does the on-call rota wear me down, as the frequency of my pro-rata on-calls means that I still enjoy doing them, even the nights!

There is a lot of paperwork involved in organizing flexible training and this continues through each post and every annual assessment. It is very important to discuss your training with your educational supervisor and to produce a Personal Learning Plan, and to get your proposed timetable (for each post within the same Trust) prospectively approved. That way, when the sarcastic comments are made about flexible trainees being 'part-time' in terms of their commitment, you will know (and have the paperwork to prove) that the reverse is true. And it is worth acknowledging that not everyone in hospital medicine will respect your choice to train in this way, but these comments are uncommon and I can count on the fingers of one hand the number I have received over the past 7 years.

As well as being an organized individual and one prepared to sift through the necessary paperwork, flexible trainees are good at multitasking – if you are not already good at this, you soon will be. There is no other way to manage a household with youngsters and to perform well on the wards. Not to mention carry out audit, complete assessments in the workplace, write the odd paper and complete your quota of on-calls!

I have been asked if I feel a sense of guilt that I can do neither job 'properly'. Honestly, for the most part I do not feel this way, but that may just be because I don't have enough time to stop and reflect. There are certainly times when I feel that I have missed out on parts of my children's childhood, my son's first school sports day for example, but I think I am much more aware of these moments missed than they are. I do think that I appreciate the time I spend with them more because it is not an everyday occurrence. Now that my son is at school, my daughter and I enjoy 'girlie' days together, which has been a real opportunity for us to bond as she is used to sharing me with her big brother.

Generally speaking, I think I have one of the best jobs there can be. I really enjoy medicine and love the time I spend with patients and their families, but I'm also able to spend more than half my time with my children, and I feel I have the best of both worlds. My time is rarely my own, but I'm happy that this is my choice and once both my children are at school and I'm no longer required 24 hours a day my free time will return. I genuinely believe that I am able to bring certain skills and experiences to my work as a direct result of being a parent and working part-time.

PERSONAL VIEW   *Tim Brabants*

From first gaining a place at Nottingham University Medical School I knew my career path was likely to be a little unconventional. I was heavily involved in the sport of sprint kayak racing and knew this was something I wanted to continue in parallel with medical training. Nottingham was really my only choice of university as it is the location of the National Watersports Centre and has a good kayak club locally. The difficulty is that training for my sport requires around 18 sessions per week, on the water, in the gym, running, swimming or cycling, and on top of this were winter training camps abroad and racing trips during the summer.

In 1996 when I started medical school I had just missed out qualifying for the Olympic Games. The first 2 years at university taught me even more about time management, trying to fit in training before and after lectures as well as finding time to study and pass exams. Social life took a massive back seat! The long holiday periods enabled me to go abroad on the training camps and I could fit in the racing trips with minimal disruption. The difficulty came in the third year when holiday times were reduced and this coincided with the Olympic qualifying year. I managed to keep on top of passing exams while training hard. My medical student housemates were essential in this process as they always made sure I knew when deadlines were and put up with my constant tiredness and occasional grumpiness.

After qualifying for the Sydney Olympics in the summer of 1999 I had the problem of how I was going to manage the fourth year with only 4 weeks off over the whole year. Luckily the Dean at the time was very keen on sport and agreed to allow me to split my fourth year over 2 years. This allowed 3 months off over the winter to spend warm weather training, then 6 months off over the build-up to the Games and time off after. This flexibility proved invaluable when I came home from Sydney with a bronze medal, Britain's first ever Olympic medal in sprint kayaking history.

It was rather strange after all the post-Olympic hype and media coverage to then return to medical school in the year below, not knowing anyone but most people knowing who I was! I made new friends and with continued support from them I was successful in completing the final 18 months of medical school and ended up graduating in the summer of 2002. I also become European Champion in the same year.

Fortunately, the NHS flexible careers scheme was just being started as I graduated. Nottingham City Hospital took me on to work as a PRHO one day a

(continued)

(*Continued*)

week for the next 2 years in the build-up to the Athens Olympics in 2004. This was an excellent opportunity to keep my hand in on the medical side of things and increase the volume of training for my sport. If I went away on a training camp, I could make up the work missed by working 2 days a week for a while. The flexibility was excellent and I was basically an extra pair of hands on either the surgical or medical assessment units, normally on Mondays, the busiest day.

My second Olympics was a little disappointing. I broke the world record in the heat but only managed fifth place in the final. After that my career took priority for the first time in 8 years. I became a full-time PRHO in Nottingham for a year in order to gain full registration with the General Medical Council. Following this I moved to Jersey for a 6-month A&E post as an SHO, with the aim of gaining further experience to enable me to do some locum work when yes, I went back to paddling full-time!

On returning to my sport, I found I was going faster than ever and think working full-time for 18 months was actually the rest my body needed. The Beijing Olympics was my next target as I felt I still had not achieved the results I was capable of. The build-up went very well with the entire focus on my training and very little on my career. This proved successful when I returned from Beijing with Gold and Bronze medals. After loads of exciting post-Olympic engagements and revelry, it was time to take my medical career seriously again. I was again lucky to receive great support from Queens Medical Centre consultants in the acute medical and emergency departments. I worked voluntarily in both these areas for a few months while being casually assessed for competence before successfully applying for a training post on the East Midlands Acute Common Care Stem programme with the view to specializing in emergency medicine. I used funding available from my sport to complete an advanced life support course prior to returning to work and thoroughly enjoyed another 18 months in full-time work during which time I also did a lot of work as a trackside doctor at Donington Park, including at the MotoGP event which was an amazing experience.

At this time I thought I was ready to focus entirely on my medical career but the call of the London Olympics was too great and so I reluctantly have had to turn away from medicine again to focus on full-time sport. I've loved my unconventional career path and could not have done it without the support from many people. After the 2012 Olympics it really will be retirement from that level of competition and back to medicine for good. Most of the people I started medical school with are now taking up registrar posts and doing really well. I'll catch up eventually!

Chapter 17 **Life as a doctor**

Five years of hard graft and multiple examinations and you finally have the honour of changing all your bank cards so that they read Dr! Some may say this is pretentious but most would think you have deserved it. Have the previous 5 years fully prepared you for the next few months of your life? Although you will have gained theoretical knowledge, you will still be lacking the practical skills and experience to be fully confident in your new job. Reading about and understanding an illness in a book is very different to seeing it in real life, especially if the patient is acutely unwell. Most graduates do find the transition from medical student to qualified doctor difficult. Do not worry – all junior doctors have been through this and most have continued in their chosen career.

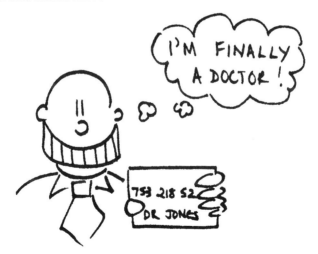

You may have the honour of changing all your bank cards so that they read Dr!

The Essential Guide to Becoming a Doctor, 3rd edition. © Adrian Blundell, Richard Harrison and Benjamin Turney. Published 2011 by Blackwell Publishing Ltd.

17.1 Foundation Year 1

Following graduation a medical student becomes a Foundation Year 1 (FY1) doctor. It is a common misconception that the term 'junior doctor' refers only to your first year following graduation. A junior doctor is in fact any doctor in a training post, which with MMC (Modernizing Medical Careers) will mean any doctor in the foundation or specialty training grades. Application for foundation jobs takes place during the autumn of the final year of medical school and the process is discussed in Chapter 15. A successful graduate is eligible for provisional registration with the General Medical Council (GMC) which lasts for 12 months. These appointments should be well supervised, but there can still be a great variety in the number of hours worked, intensity of work, training provision and level of senior support. It is therefore worth spending some time researching the potential post, especially if it is in a hospital or area of the country where you have not worked. At a minimum, visit the hospital and talk to staff who are already employed by that Trust. The work involved with each post will also vary depending on the specialty. Some may involve less out-of-hours commitment (e.g. general practice, psychiatry) but bear in mind this will mean a lower wage. There could also be great variety in the amount of responsibility and support given.

The first day

The FY1 posts commence on the first Wednesday of August. Each hospital should run an induction course for the new doctors. For FY1 posts, the induction will often be on the day prior to commencing work so there are at least some junior doctors available for duty on the first Wednesday. The inductions vary between hospitals but will include a variety of lectures and small group work. The topics covered will include hospital orientation, hospital computer systems including log in and passwords, the process for requesting tests, accommodation and pay, car parking, and dealing with death and the coroner. There will be a great deal of paperwork that will need to be completed, with the most important form being that of your bank details, so you get paid.

Things to organize by your first day (or soon after)

- GMC registration
- Indemnity insurance: this covers you from a legal point in the event of mistakes. Limited cover is provided by the NHS establishment employing you but it is ESSENTIAL to take out extra cover with an organization such as the Medical Defence Union or Medical Protection Society

- Pay roll
- Accommodation and car parking
- ID badge and computer access
- Copy of work rota, to enable essential swaps asap
- Hepatitis B immunity
- Criminal Record Bureau certificate

After induction and sorting out the paperwork, it is time to pick up your bleep/pager, find the wards and your team. Teams of doctors in hospitals are referred to as a 'firm' and traditionally consisted of one to two consultants, a specialist registrar (SpR) and some senior house officers (SHOs) and JHOs (possibly one or two), with each firm responsible for patients under their care. With the advent of MMC, the firms will consist of FY1 and FY2 doctors and then trainees at various stages of their specialist training. There may be little in the way of formal induction to the ward – straight in at the deep end! However, you should have had a chance to undertake shadowing experience with your predecessor, so it won't all be new. Rather than working as part of one firm, doctors tend to work in bigger teams, enabling absence through leave or on-call commitments in order to have less impact on the day-to-day running of the ward.

17.2 Life as a foundation doctor

As a qualified doctor, the hospital staff will now treat you a little differently. While a medical student it is easy to feel in the way and a spare part, but once qualified your skills will be much in demand. There will be support around, especially during the first few weeks and usually someone more senior from whom advice may be sought. The first few days can be daunting but will no doubt pass quickly. You will wonder where all the knowledge from medical school has gone and why most of it is no longer relevant. The theoretical information has been taught and now it is time to put it into practice – you can only really learn how to become a junior doctor by performing the job itself. This is when you will start wishing you had spent even more of your student days in the hospital. The transition from being a senior medical student to once again being at the bottom of the chain of command can also be difficult, especially for mature students. As an FY1 doctor, you need to take instruction from your senior colleagues and certainly the majority of the job can be mundane, involving a great deal of chasing results and ordering investigations. It is essential to become competent at the basics before progressing, hence the introduction of MMC. It is important to realize that you are an important member of the team. Being a good foundation trainee involves excellent organization, communication and team-working skills. You are not expected to have an exhaustive knowledge and it is imperative to know your own limits and ask for help appropriately. Knowing your patients' medical history and management thoroughly not only impresses your seniors but will also help improve your enjoyment of the job.

Medical jobs

The junior doctors are responsible for the patients under the care of their consultant. The consultant will perform a ward round once or twice a week with the rest of the firm. It is the foundation doctors' responsibility to know who and where the patients are and to be able to tell the other members of the team the reason for admission, the medical history and relevant investigations that have been performed. A management plan will be made for each patient and, following the ward round, all the jobs must be performed. This will involve chasing and ordering tests, and performing practical procedures. If, during the admission, any patients become unwell, then the nurses will contact the doctor via the pager for review. The bleep, although initially a novelty, will soon become hated.

Surgical jobs

The luxury of a 9 a.m. start will not be afforded in surgery – surgical ward rounds tend to start at 8 a.m. The ward round is when a senior surgical doctor will do a tour of all the firm's patients at this time; the consultant will usually attend just two or three of these per week. After the ward round, it is again the job of the foundation doctor to order tests and chase results. During the week there will be sessions called pre-clerking. This is where patients are seen the week before their routine operation and bloods can be taken and other tests performed. At this time it can be checked that the patient is fit enough for the operation and an anaesthetic opinion can be sought if necessary. The rest of the week involves looking after and treating patients who are at pre- and post-operation stage.

Other jobs

As previously mentioned, at least a couple of posts during the Foundation Programme will be in medical and surgical specialties. In view of the variety of posts on offer, the potential options for jobs in the Foundation Programme is almost endless and in some ways depends on whether certain departments want to develop training for junior doctors in their specialties. The smaller the specialty, the fewer posts available for foundation doctors. Study the application site for the options.

On-call

A hospital must be open, and emergency healthcare provided, 24 hours a day, and hence the doctor's working day is not 9 to 5. To provide this 'after hours' medical care, each day there will be a team of doctors on-call (on-take) for each specialty. It is their responsibility to admit patients who are referred to the hospital from either casualty or general practitioners. The term 'on-call' has been traditionally used because most of the rotas worked in hospital were of the on-call variety. With the changes in working practice, many rotas are no longer on-call, but for ease of describing out-of-hours work this term continues to be used.

The foundation trainee tends to be the first doctor to see the patient when he or she arrives at the hospital. This involves taking a history (asking relevant questions), performing examinations and investigations, and attempting to diagnose and treat the patient. During or immediately after the on-call period, the more senior doctors will perform a 'post-take' ward round where further management plans can be made. If an acutely unwell patient is admitted, then it is sometimes more appropriate to seek senior help early and initiate treatment immediately.

A further responsibility while on-call is to look after the patients on the wards, known as ward cover. Out of hours there will only be one or two doctors responsible for the medical care of all the hospital inpatients. Again the jobs will vary from reviewing sick patients to looking up results and performing practical procedures. Depending on the specialty, on-call could involve either admitting patients, ward cover, or both.

Unfortunately, life as a junior doctor is not quite as glamorous as it is portrayed in many medical dramas; indeed, much of the work can be fairly boring, for example looking up blood results and writing them up in notes. Nevertheless, there will be times when you are dealing with very poorly patients who need urgent medical attention, and there is no better feeling than when you have initiated treatment and seen a patient improve. On the downside there will also be times when patients die despite all the intervention that you have attempted. Most of a junior doctor's work is essentially clerking but there will be bursts of fear and adrenaline. Although most of the time support will be near, there could be occasions when you are the only doctor around and it will be necessary to think and act quickly. It is important to be able to work as a team member and liaise and delegate with other staff to perform the necessary tasks. It is easy to say, but it will be essential to keep a cool head, and in most circumstances it will be possible to think first and act later. Roughly translated, take a step back and think about the situation, rather than rushing in and doing something that could be potentially dangerous. And if in doubt, look to one of the experienced nurses for advice – they can be your best friend or your worst enemy!

Remember that a foundation doctor will often be the initial contact for patients, relatives and other healthcare professionals, so appearance, good communication skills, and bedside manner are essential attributes.

Things to consider as a junior doctor

- Be friendly and smile
- Take your breaks and organize holiday leave early
- Be reliable
- Call for help sooner rather than later – your seniors do not like surprises!
- Have interests outside medicine and enjoy your free time
- Never shout at colleagues
- Prepare for the future

Cardiac arrests

It is important as a doctor to keep a cool head and, as mentioned previously, for the majority of scenarios it will be possible to take a step back and consider a management plan. However, one situation where urgent action is required is in the event of a cardiac arrest. This means that a patient's heart has stopped. Each hospital will have a team of doctors who are on-call to cover such emergencies – surprisingly these doctors are often fairly junior and most foundation trainees will find themselves involved at some point.

When your shift begins, you will be handed the 'cardiac arrest' bleep from a colleague, who will no doubt tell tales of horror from the previous shift. Unlike your everyday pager, the cardiac arrest bleep lets out a series of ear-piercing tones, often followed closely by a voice telling you where the emergency is located. As a newly qualified doctor, you will certainly have a great deal of anxiety related to carrying this bleep and will experience a sudden adrenaline surge when it actually sounds. The idea is to then run to the appropriate ward, although the initial feeling is to walk slowly in the opposite direction, hoping other more senior people will arrive first. We will not discuss actual management of these situations but advise that it is still important to try to keep a cool head, think logically and elect a team leader to help guide the staff. To help with managing these emergencies, most doctors are offered the opportunity to take part in an advanced life support course, which will run through real-life situations with mannequins. Although also a little nerve wracking, these courses can be good fun and of course the patients can always be resuscitated!

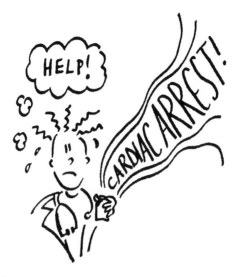

Life as a junior doctor

Communication skills

One of the most important skills to be gained during your student days (and beyond) is the ability to be a good communicator. Unfortunately, this has not always been reflected in the medical school course. In fact many of the complaints from patients and relatives (and indeed other medical personnel) are a direct result of a breakdown in communication. Firstly, it is necessary to explain to your patient (and relatives if appropriate) about any information as it becomes available. Medical jargon should be avoided and explanations pitched to the level appropriate to your patient (but don't patronize). It is essential that doctors and other medical personnel involved in the care of the patient liaise with each other regarding diagnoses, test results, information relayed to patients, etc. Documentation in notes is crucial since, in the age of increasing litigation, this will probably be the only evidence available – it is not guaranteed that a doctor will remember the events a year later (or even the specific patient). Occasionally, mistakes may happen and patients and/or relatives will be unhappy with situations. Apologize if necessary and always remember that honesty is the best policy.

Accommodation

Until 2009, accommodation on the hospital site was routinely provided for first-year doctors, free of charge. With the advent of the European Working Time Directive and reduction in hours, this is no longer the case.

Pay

After 5 years of poverty, the first wage packet will be a great comfort. The only problem is that the majority of the content will be spent paying off the debts built up over the last few years. A supplement to your income will be cremation form fees: when a patient dies a cremation form must be completed and signed by the doctor to permit the cremation to proceed. This is a legal document and, like any other legal document in medicine, a fee is charged. Just don't forget to tell the tax man!

17.3 Specialist training

As doctors progress up the career ladder, their duties can change. With seniority comes increased responsibility and decision-making. The advent of reduction in hours and the introduction of MMC could see junior doctors becoming less experienced. There is also a call for more senior doctors to have greater hands-on contact with patients. For this reason some junior doctors still find frustration with their work when they still have to 'run things by the boss'. No matter what grade, there will still be laborious tasks to complete but in general there will be greater exposure to more complex patients and also more complicated procedures. During specialist training, most doctors will be required to study for postgraduate diplomas. It can be difficult to juggle clinical commitments and family life during this time, so good time management will be essential. It is not uncommon for doctors to take several attempts to get through these exams, which then also adds a financial burden as the cost has to be met personally. In fact this could often be the first time an exam has been failed during a medic's life, which can be hard to accept by some. Try not to be disheartened – it is often no reflection on your ability as a clinician.

Three or four years post graduation is also a time when some doctors decide to change their career path. By this stage they have had a chance to think more carefully about their future career and have had more experience of the different specialties. The change is often due to lifestyle decisions, family commitments, disillusionment with a particular career or difficult career progression due to competition.

17.4 Senior medical appointments

So 4–6 years of undergraduate medicine and multiple exams, followed by up to 12 years of postgraduate training and further exams, and you have finally made it, an independent practitioner! So surely now it is all about sports cars, large houses and ultimate power – who would question such a knowledgeable specialist. The reality is unfortunately different. Although doctors will earn a comfortable wage, few will earn the big bucks without a large private practice. There are still considerable aspects of the job that can be routine and there has been an increased amount of paperwork introduced. Of course a greater proportion of the work will involve managerial aspects, education and dealing with the politics involved in running departments and practices. Another fairly recent change is the necessity for continuing medical education. Medicine is such a rapidly advancing field that it is essential that all doctors show they are keeping up to date. This will involve continuing research and attending various meetings and conferences and may even involve the introduction of further assessments. Hopefully, though, a doctor will have chosen the particular specialty due to a keen interest and therefore in general will be enjoying the work.

17.5 Regulation of doctors

The future regulation of doctors is currently under review, with implementation of several important changes commencing in 2010. There have been several high-profile cases in the news that have led to a need to tighten regulation of doctors and ultimately improve patient safety. One of these cases was that of Harold Shipman, a GP working in the Manchester region who was found guilty of killing 15 of his patients in 2000.

Prior to discussing the implications and organization of revalidation, it is worth mentioning two regulatory bodies. The GMC was established in 1858 and its main purpose is to 'protect, promote and maintain the health and safety of the public by ensuring proper standards in the practice of medicine'. In reality this equates to keeping a register of qualified doctors, encouraging good medical practice, promoting high standards of medical education and dealing with doctors who underperform.

The Postgraduate Medical Education and Training Board (PMETB) was created in 2003 as a non-governmental independent body to formalize and oversee postgraduate medical education. Its main roles are in approving all postgraduate training programmes and certifying doctors who have completed their training.

In April 2010 the PMETB and GMC merged. This new body will now be responsible for medical education right through from undergraduate to postgraduate level and beyond. And 2009 saw the introduction of licences to practice; a doctor who wishes to work now not only needs to register with the GMC but also apply for a licence. Following the introduction of this, a further system called revalidation will be introduced; this will require doctors to renew their licence to practice every 5 years. In order for a renewal to be granted, doctors will need to provide evidence that they are up to date and fit to practice.

17.6 Difficult times

In general the majority of doctors enjoy most of their working time. It is common to experience difficult times but these are often transient. There will be times when stress levels are high and this is particularly the case when patients die, especially if unexpected. The responsibility and demands of the job can lead to exhaustion, especially with increasing litigation, complaints and patients' expectations. It is important to talk to colleagues and friends and consider having a debriefing session following difficult clinical scenarios. If feedback is not forthcoming from senior colleagues, then arrange a time to sit down with the bosses and discuss your progress. It may even be necessary to take some leave or have a break from medicine. It is also essential to keep active interests outside medicine. Whatever difficulties you are experiencing, someone will have been through the same scenario so seek help early and try not to bottle up feelings.

17.7 Summary

For many, the first year post graduation is both the best and worst year of their lives. After a gruelling 5 years at medical school, you are finally earning money and hopefully making a difference. For many the glory and the glamour are not as they had imagined and the routine, sometimes boring, jobs are not stimulating. Comments such as 'A monkey could be trained to do my job' are not very encouraging for future doctors. In defence of the hospitals, many have introduced new methods to try to reduce the long hours worked by the doctors and, in doing so, have cut down on some of the more laborious tasks that would not be classed as being educational and so not suitable for a training doctor. Nevertheless, a great majority of the work as a junior doctor will be routine, but the skills gained in the first couple of years are essential to a future career in any of the specialties. Like many professions, it is necessary to be an apprentice for some part of your training and, after all, it only lasts a short time.

  This chapter has tried to give an honest view of the reality of being a doctor. Remember that the majority of doctors succeed in their chosen specialty and have enjoyable careers. The job of a doctor has great variety and is very rewarding. Always want the best for your patients and try not to get too demoralized with the Government using the NHS as a political tool and the obvious financial implications of this.

PERSONAL VIEW *Pip Parson*

Wow! You're a 'doctor', a word you probably never realistically thought would apply to you. The shiny exciting feeling after graduation is starting to dull and that awesome once-in-a-lifetime tan from the long summer holiday and distant memories of the 2 weeks shadowing are also beginning to fade. Suddenly it begins to dawn on you that with that title comes real responsibility.

The first few days of starting work are like any new attachment – an induction full of boring lectures and reams of confusing paperwork. It's hard to concentrate when you haven't seen your mates for ages and all you really want to know is how many weekends you are going to give up, how much you are getting paid and, most of all, when you can get on to the wards to start saving lives. Compared with most, I had been fairly diligent during shadowing, learning to navigate the wards and trying to befriend and memorize the names of the nurses who, as I soon found out, knew far more about how to look after the stroke patients than I did. Still, my greatest fear was realized when all the coloured boxes on the rota confirmed that I was 'FY1 of the day' on the first weekend. Glamorous as that sounds, it actually meant that I was due to cover all the medical wards, doing any jobs needed and being at the beck and call of all the nurses if there was anything at all going wrong. (Remember what I said about making friends with them from the beginning to make your life easier!) The weekend shift lasts for 13 hours on Saturday and Sunday with only the help of one SHO who didn't start until 11 a.m., leaving me alone for 3 hours. Worse still, true to rota coordinator traditions, the SHO covering with me was a locum, as yet to be appointed.

I turned up early, heading to the Acute Medical Unit, aware that somewhere I had to locate the 'blue folder' that contained all the jobs like blood tests and patient reviews that needed doing over the weekend. A helpful SHO had advised me that I should first find the elusive folder and then head straight to the mess for a cup of tea and start prioritizing, as it would probably be the only chance I'd get to sit down all day. I was stopped on the way before I had even taken off my coat by a senior nurse saying 'Are you the junior on call? I've been bleeping you for ages. There's a man with coffee-ground vomit on ward 5 who needs reviewing.' Looking through the folder and finding several pages of jobs from each of the wards and my bleep going off before I even had a chance to look through them, it felt like a nightmare before it had even begun. I arrived on the ward, immediately swarmed upon with cries

(continued)

(Continued)

of 'Thank goodness! The doctor's here!' It made me want to look around, hoping that they weren't actually referring to me. I had been warned to be sceptical when told that a patient has coffee-ground vomit because 'it's usually an exaggeration and just a ploy to get you to respond to the bleep faster'. As it turned out, this patient didn't look very well at all and stared at me frightened before clearly demonstrating textbook haematemesis (vomiting blood) all over the bed right in front of me. I was horrified and unsure if I should jump straight for the crash button in panic. I reasoned that the team probably wouldn't be too impressed with me and I should attempt to do something first, but what? All sensible thought seemed to have vacated my head and despite what I was feeling, I managed to put on what I think was a calm exterior and asked the nurse to repeat the observations (pulse and blood pressure) to buy me some time to look up the management in my little handbook – oxygen, BP, intravenous fluids, blood. Obviously, I knew this. Looking back at the patient, I still felt unnerved. After 10 minutes of more vomiting and a blood pressure that was worryingly low, I had reached my threshold and was about to grab the phone when miraculously a smiling SHO wandered onto the ward offering her assistance. With her support and a little perspective, everything seemed so much simpler. I realized that although I would have ultimately needed senior assistance, the initial basic management had been do-able.

So my first weekend did feel rather traumatic, but rather than painting a scene of complete doom and gloom, it did set me up well for the year ahead. Often situations that are initially a cue to panic seem a lot simpler if you just stand back, take a breath and work through things logically. It will be an extremely rare occurrence if you find yourself completely alone; as is always drummed into you, call for help early as no one expects (or wants) you to be a hero!

Moving through the different FY1 rotations, there are always new things expected of you, like running the surgical ward rounds on your own because your whole team have gone to theatre *again*, or turning up at pre-op clinic where patients get assessed for their anaesthetic risk prior to surgery and finding out that you're on your own and that all these people coming to see 'the doctor' are just there to see *you*. The most important thing I learnt that makes a real difference to being a 'good FY1' to work with or not is organization. It is the key to all things FY1. Life is much easier if it is a skill that you master early on and you will reap the rewards for it, whether this is getting to go home on time or having seniors on your side who are more likely to help out with 'silly' questions or offer opportunities to have a go at new things.

At first, everything feels difficult, but by the end of the year you'll find that perhaps things really weren't so bad and you wonder what all the stress was about. The best thing about the work is that it is nearly always interesting and you really do learn new things every day.

Chapter 18 **Career options**

It is unusual for prospective medical students to know what their ultimate specialty will be. Of those who think they do know, most subsequently change their minds. By the end of medical school the majority of students have a general idea of the broad area of medicine they wish to continue in (e.g. general practice, hospital medicine). Graduating from university with a medical degree allows a diverse range of possible career opportunities to suit people with all types of personalities and interests. Unfortunately, some medical graduates are not actually aware of all the possibilities available. This may be due to the small size of certain specialties and the lack of coverage during the medical school curriculum. It is essential to be aware of the options and prospects before embarking on postgraduate training and although not intended to be exhaustive, we hope this chapter outlines the majority of choices. With the changes in medical training, there are still areas of uncertainty with regard to length of training and progression. It will be worthwhile reviewing the individual specialty websites (see Table 18.1) for up-to-date information. The statistical information used in this chapter can be found on the Department of Health's website. For more information we recommend reading the BMA's guide to career choice (found on their website), the book *So You Want To Be a Brain Surgeon?* (Oxford University Press) and the website www.medicalcareers.nhs.uk.

18.1 The career ladder

The generic career ladder has been described in Chapter 15. All doctors will enter foundation training for 2 years following university. If successful they will then embark on specialist training in either a run-through grade or via fixed-year appointments. The number of years spent during run-through

The Essential Guide to Becoming a Doctor, 3rd edition. © Adrian Blundell,
Richard Harrison and Benjamin Turney. Published 2011 by Blackwell Publishing Ltd.

will depend on the specialty chosen (approximately 5–8 years). Some doctors will also spend time studying for a higher degree, which will mean an extra 2 years for an MD or 3 years for a PhD. Each rung of the ladder will need to be successfully completed in order to progress. This could involve completion of certain exams or assessments and will always involve attainment of the competencies set out by each specialty which will be reviewed at an annual ARCP (Annual Review of Competence Progression) meeting. The majority of doctors become GPs, with the next two largest specialties being medicine and surgery. For this reason there are separate chapters outlining the training in these (Chapters 19–21). The table below summarizes the number of doctors working at different grades in the UK in 2005.

	1995	2005
GPs	28 869	35 302
Consultants	19 524	31 993
Registrar level	11 466	18 006
SHO level	13 342	21 642
PRHO/F1 level	3 298	4 663
All NHS doctors	84 459	122 345

The total figure in the table includes other groups of doctors, for example staff grades, associate specialists and dental practitioners. There has been a steady increase in recruitment over the last 10 years, although with the current financial climate it is unlikely this progression will continue, and more worryingly there is actually talk of doctors losing their jobs or retiring doctors not being replaced. As of 2005, 26% of consultants and 55% of F1s were female, demonstrating the increased number of female places at medical school but the general lack of female senior hospital clinicians.

18.2 The choices

A major advantage to having a medical degree is the large number of possible career options available. Choosing a particular path requires considerable thought as it can have a huge impact on a doctor's eventual professional and personal life. The choice will depend on an individual's personality and interests. It is necessary for a doctor to decide what he or she eventually wants to get out of the job and the level of responsibility and commitment desired in the future. It is also essential to think about the career many years down the line as personal aspects will change, for example family commitments. Other factors to consider include the amount of patient contact, opportunities for research, flexible working arrangements, ease of taking time out, individual interests, number of postgraduate examinations and level of competition. During university most students will find certain subject areas that they have a greater interest in and also may meet inspirational clinicians during their education. Try to have a broad idea of your speciality towards graduation but avoid a definite decision too early. Currently, it is possible to change career paths, but this may become more difficult with run-through training. As well as the large number of medical choices, some graduates decide that being a doctor is not what they envisaged and they leave the profession altogether. Many other professions recognize the qualities that medical graduates possess and offer employment without it being necessary to gain a further degree. A future development could be the increased use of psychometric testing in helping a medical student or doctor choose a career. These tests are becoming more popular as an assessment to determine suitability for gaining a place a medical school.

Choosing a career: things to consider

- Competition for jobs, now and higher up the training ladder
- Amount of patient contact
- Level of responsibility
- Personality
- Possibility for research and teaching
- Opportunities for time out of training
- Opportunities for flexible training
- Out-of-hours commitment, especially at consultant level
- Balance between professional and personal life
- Job satisfaction
- Can you imagine working in this speciality for the rest of your life?

18.3 The options

These can be divided broadly into general practice or medical specialties (community or hospital based), as summarized in Table 18.1. Remember other options such as joining the armed forces, being a doctor on board a cruise ship, working in rural areas in other countries, voluntary work in areas of need, or working in non-NHS environments such as the pharmaceutical industry, medical journalism or medical law. All hospital specialties require at least one postgraduate qualification. The timing of these exams varies between subjects and will certainly change with Modernizing Medical Careers. Currently, some specialties actually require a postgraduate diploma before entering registrar level training; for example for haematology, MRCP

Table 18.1 Summary of the specialties available and the postgraduate examinations necessary

Specialty	Run-through training?	Parent specialty	Subspecialty	Useful information	Postgraduate qualification
Emergency medicine	No	A&E	Paediatric emergency medicine	www.collemergencymed.ac.uk	MCEM
Allergy	No	Medicine		www.jchmt.org.uk/allergy	MRCP
Anaesthetics	No	Anaesthetics		www.rcoa.ac.uk	FRCAnaes
Audiological medicine	No	Medicine		www.jchmt.org.uk/audio	MRCP or equivalent
Cardiology	No	Medicine	Stroke medicine	www.jchmt.org.uk/cardio	MRCP
Cardiothoracic surgery	No	Surgery		www.jcst.org www.rcseng.ac.uk www.iscp.ac.uk	MRCS
Chemical pathology (clinical biochemistry)	Yes	Pathology	Metabolic medicine	www.rcpath.org	MRCPath
Child and adolescent psychiatry	No	Psychiatry		www.rcpsych.ac.uk	MRCPsych
Clinical cytogenics and molecular genetics	No	Pathology		www.rcpath.org	MRCPath
Clinical genetics	No	Medicine		www.jchmt.org.uk/clingen	MRCP
Clinical neurophysiology	No	Medicine		www.jchmt.org.uk/clinneuro	MRCP
Clinical oncology	No	Medicine		www.rcr.ac.uk	FRCR
Clinical pharmacology and therapeutics	No	Medicine	Stroke medicine	www.jchmt.org.uk/clinpharm	MRCP
Clinical radiology	Yes	Radiology		www.rcr.ac.uk	FRCR
Dermatology	No	Medicine		www.jchmt.org.uk/dermat	MRCP
Endocrinology	No	Medicine	Diabetology	www.jchmt.org.uk/endocrin	MRCP
Forensic psychiatry	No	Psychiatry		www.rcpsych.ac.uk	MRCPsych

(continued)

Table 18.1 (*Continued*)

Specialty	Run-through training?	Parent specialty	Subspecialty	Useful information	Postgraduate qualification
Gastroenterology	No	Medicine	Hepatology	www.jchmt.org.uk/gastro	MRCP
General (internal) medicine	No	Medicine	Acute, metabolic and stroke medicine	www.jchmt.org.uk/gim	MRCP
General practice	Yes	General practice		www.rcgp.org.uk	MRCGP
General psychiatry	No	Psychiatry	Liaison and substance misuse psychiatry	www.rcpsych.ac.uk	MRCPsych
General surgery	No	Surgery		www.jcst.org www.rcseng.ac.uk www.iscp.ac.uk	MRCS
Genitourinary medicine	No	Medicine		www.jchmt.org.uk/gum	MRCP
Geriatric medicine	No	Medicine	Stroke medicine	www.jchmt.org.uk/geriat	MRCP
Haematology	No	Medicine		www.jchmt.org.uk/haem	MRCPath
Histopathology	Yes	Pathology	Cytopathology, forensic pathology, neuropathology, paediatric pathology	www.rcpath.org	MRCPath
Immunology	No	Medicine		www.jchmt.org.uk/immun	MRCP
Infectious diseases	No	Medicine		www.jchmt.org.uk/infect	MRCP
Intensive care	No	Anaesthetics		www.rcoa.ac.uk	FRCAnaes
Medical microbiology	Yes	Pathology		www.rcpath.org	MRCPath
Medical oncology	No	Medicine		www.jchmt.org.uk/medonc	MRCP
Medical ophthalmology	No	Medicine		www.jchmt.org.uk/ophthal	MRCP
Neurology	No	Medicine	Stroke medicine	www.jchmt.org.uk/neuro	MRCP
Neurosurgery	Yes	Surgery		www.jcst.org www.rcseng.ac.uk www.iscp.ac.uk	MRCS

Specialty		Related area	Website	Exam
Nuclear medicine	No	Medicine	www.jchmt.org.uk/nuclear	MRCP/FRCR
Obstetrics and gynaecology	Yes	Obstetrics and gynaecology	www.rcog.org.uk	MRCOG
		Gynaecological oncology, maternal and fetal medicine, reproductive medicine, sexual and reproductive health, urogynaecology		
Occupational medicine	No	Medicine	www.facoccmed.ac.uk	AFOM
Old age psychiatry	No	Psychiatry	www.rcpsych.ac.uk	MRCPsych
Ophthalmology	Yes	Ophthalmology	www.rcophth.ac.uk	FRCOphth
Oral and maxillofacial surgery	No	Dentistry/Surgery	www.rcseng.ac.uk/dental	MRCS
Otolaryngology (ENT)	No	Surgery	www.jcst.org www.rcseng.ac.uk www.iscp.ac.uk	MRCS
Paediatric cardiology	No	Surgery	www.jcst.org www.rcseng.ac.uk www.iscp.ac.uk	MRCS
Paediatric surgery	No	Surgery	www.jcst.org www.rcseng.ac.uk www.iscp.ac.uk	MRCS
Paediatrics	Yes	Paediatrics	www.rcpch.ac.uk	MRCPaeds
		Community child health, neonatal medicine and specialties by organ system		
Palliative medicine	No	Medicine	www.jchmt.org.uk/palliative	MRCP
Pharmaceutical medicine	No	Medicine	www.jchmt.org.uk/pharma	MRCP
Plastic surgery	No	Surgery	www.jcst.org www.rcseng.ac.uk www.iscp.ac.uk	MRCS

(continued)

Table 18.1 (Continued)

Specialty	Run-through training?	Parent specialty	Subspecialty	Useful information	Postgraduate qualification
Psychiatry of learning disability	No	Psychiatry		www.rcpsych.ac.uk	MRCPsych
Psychotherapy	No	Psychiatry		www.rcpsych.ac.uk	MRCPsych
Public health medicine	Yes	Public health medicine		www.fph.org.uk	MFPH
Rehabilitation medicine	No	Medicine	Stroke medicine	www.jchmt.org.uk/rehab	MRCP
Renal medicine	No	Medicine		www.jchmt.org.uk/renal	MRCP
Respiratory medicine	No	Medicine		www.jchmt.org.uk/respir	MRCP
Rheumatology	No	Medicine		www.jchmt.org.uk/rheum	MRCP
Trauma and orthopaedic surgery	Yes	Surgery		www.jcst.org www.rcseng.ac.uk www.iscp.ac.uk	MRCS
Tropical medicine	No	Medicine		www.jchmt.org.uk/infect	MRCP
Urology	No	Surgery		www.jcst.org www.rcseng.ac.uk www.iscp.ac.uk	MRCS

Table 18.2 Number of doctors working in each specialty as of 2005

Specialty	Consultant grade	Registrar grade	Female consultants
A&E	689	711	151 (22%)
Anaesthetics	4502	2221	1241 (28%)
Clinical oncology	438	281	159 (36%)
Dental	671	345	148 (22%)
General medicine group	7072	4155	1634 (23%)
Obstetrics and gynaecology	1458	1290	432 (30%)
Paediatrics	2033	1617	843 (41%)
Pathology	2398	966	852 (36%)
Public health	927	252	425 (46%)
Psychiatry	3759	1032	1372 (36%)
Radiology	2058	935	620 (30%)
Surgery	5988	4201	476 (8%)
All	31 993	18 006	8353 (26%)

(Member of the Royal College of Physicians) is required during broad-based medical training and then MRCPath (Member of the Royal College of Pathologists) needs to be passed during the haematology specialization. Although not compulsory, most GPs will complete the MRCGP. More confusingly, some specialties offer run-through training (from the end of Foundation Programme to completion of training) and others have a second stage of competitive entry after 2 or 3 core training years. Table 18.2 shows the number of doctors working in each specialty as of 2005.

Emergency medicine

As the name suggests, doctors in the emergency department (ED) see patients who have a medical emergency or some form of accident. This can range from life-threatening conditions including major trauma to injuries from minor accidents. Some of these patients will have been taken to the department by emergency ambulance but many with more minor problems present themselves. Patients in the ED are triaged (assessed by a nurse to be seen in order of priority) so that the more unwell patients are dealt with first. Traditionally, there used to be long waiting times in British EDs before patients with minor ailments were seen. The introduction of the Government's 4-hour maximum wait target has put increased pressure on the workforce and departments may get fined if patients are waiting over this time. Working in the ED can be hectic and has an unpredictable nature as a patient with any problem could attend. Traditionally, most ED consultants were from a surgical background but the new training programme does not recognize qualifications from other specialties and all ED doctors must pass the emergency medicine exams. There is a lot of opportunity for practical procedures, especially suturing, and as many patients are transferred to other departments, good communication skills with other healthcare professionals is important. Most departments now have separate facilities for the care of children and paediatric emergency medicine is now an accredited subspecialty.

Training

Following the Foundation Programme, the new training in emergency medicine will involve 6 years of specialist training. The programme is divided into 3 years core specialty training and 3 years higher specialty training. In England, Wales and Northern Ireland entry to higher specialty training is by competitive application. Core specialty training consists of 2 years of Acute Care Common Stem (ACCS) training and 1 year of CT3 specialties. The last 3 years (specialty training years 4–6) are spent in EDs, gaining additional clinical competences, consolidating prior training and gaining skills in academic emergency medicine, critical appraisal and management topics. The examination to become a Member of the College of Emergency Medicine (MCEM) is required for progression through training.

Skills

Good team-working skills, leadership skills, common sense, able to keep a cool head under pressure, communication skills.

Advantages

Fast paced, variety of cases, opportunities to be involved as a doctor at local events, multidisciplinary, opportunities for flexible and part-time working.

Disadvantages

Little continuity of care because of the high turnover of patients, full shift rotas so more antisocial hours (more weekends and nights than most specialties), stressful.

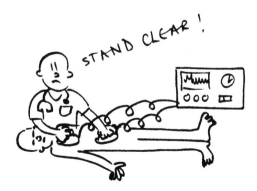

Career paths: A&E

Anaesthetics

Put simply, the anaesthetist's main job is to put patients to sleep ready for a surgical procedure and then wake them up again afterwards. Many operations are now performed under local or regional anaesthesia, which has increased the number of procedures possible. There are many other roles for an anaesthetist, including an extended role in managing pre- and post-operative care and administering pain relief, acutely in the form of epidurals and also for patients with chronic pain problems. Junior anaesthetists are often involved in helping at cardiac arrests in a hospital and will often be part of the arrest team (a team of doctors and other health professionals called immediately if a patient stops breathing). Like emergency medicine, this is another specialty with little continuity of care unless an anaesthetist has responsibility for the intensive care unit (ICU). Factors such as service provision and shift rotas mean that anaesthetics has good opportunities for flexible training. It is now quite common for a consultant to subspecialize in one field of anaesthesia, for example cardiothoracic, paediatric or intensive care. It is important to be a team player as it is necessary to deal with hospital staff from all areas, not just the operating theatres. Some of the work can be routine but emergencies can develop quickly, and so the ability to cope with stress is also essential.

Training
Foundation Programme and then 2 or 3 years of core training either in anaesthetics alone or during the early years in combination with other core acute specialty training. Some doctors have traditionally moved into anaesthesia after passing the MRCP, although this pathway is now more unlikely. Exams are a requirement of progression to the higher training in anaesthesia. The higher training is for five further years.

Skills
Good team-working skills, leadership skills, able to keep a cool head under pressure, communication skills.

Advantages
Opportunities for flexible or part-time working, wide variety of patient care, management of acutely unwell patients, great satisfaction in providing immediate life support to critically unwell patients.

Disadvantages
Minimal continuity of care as patients are handed back to hospital teams after operations or ICU admission, long operations sat at the head of the bed, unpredictable nature.

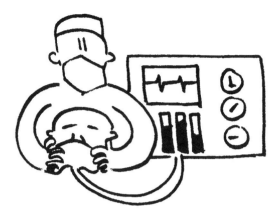

Career paths: anaesthetics

Obstetrics and gynaecology

Two specialties for the price of one! Obstetrics involves caring for pregnant women and gynaecology covers diseases of the female genital tract. It is essential to have knowledge of many medical fields, including endocrinology, medicine, neonatology, physiology and sexual problems, and also to have the relevant surgical skills. In obstetrics it is necessary to know the physiological changes during pregnancy and then have the necessary skills to perform safe deliveries. From a gynaecological aspect the caseload includes sexual problems, urological complaints, menstrual disorders and gynaecological cancers. Many students enjoy their time on the labour suite dealing with relatively young and healthy patients and also assisting in the delivery of babies. This can be a slightly skewed picture, and it is important not to forget that mothers and babies can run into problems and emotions can run high. It is essential that a doctor in this specialty can deal with stressful situations. Although possible to become a general obstetrics and gynaecology doctor, many trainees now have a subspecialty interest especially in the larger tertiary referral centres, for example gynaecological malignancy or reproductive medicine.

Training
Foundation Programme and then 7 years run-through training. MRCOG Part 1 and set competencies are required to move up to ST3 and MRCOG Part 2 and further competencies are needed to continue to the final stages of training.

Skills
Empathic, ability to work under stressful conditions, communication skills.

Advantages
Relatively young and often healthy patients, wide variety of subspecialties, emotional rewards, delivering babies.

Disadvantages
Antisocial hours even for consultants, stressful, extremely emotional if things go wrong, litigation, patients' expectations.

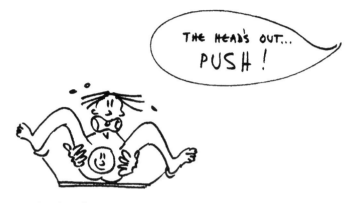

Career paths: obstetrics

Paediatrics

This is the branch of medicine providing care for children. The opportunity for subspecialization in paediatrics is more limited than in adult medicine and many of the consultants will act as general paediatric physicians. At the large tertiary referral centres there may be doctors with a special interest in certain areas. This branch of training is also followed for neonatology (care of the new-born) and community paediatrics. Many undergraduates enjoy the specialty ('Ah, babies!'), but in a similar way to obstetrics and gynaecology, emotions can run high during stressful times and remember that most of the patients will come with their parents. It is interesting that it was only fairly recently that paediatrics became independent of adult medicine with the development of its own college – prior to this the postgraduate exam was the same as for adult physicians. Opportunities for flexible training are good as can be seen by the high number of female consultants. Like obstetrics and gynaecology, this specialty is likely to require more senior input at unsocial hours.

Training
Foundation Programme 2 years followed by 8 years run-through training. Entry to ST3 requires MRCPCH Part 1A and B or equivalent and entry to ST4 requires MRCPCH or equivalent.

Skills
Don't have to be a big kid but it probably helps, calm, friendly, able to cope with potential emotional and stressful times.

Advantages
Wide variety of conditions, diagnostically challenging as history not always easy, flexible training, high cure rates.

Disadvantages
Unsocial hours even as senior doctors, emotionally draining.

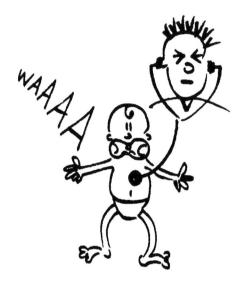

Career paths: paediatrics

Pathology

This is the study of disease processes. The image that comes to mind is the pathologist performing the autopsy (post-mortem) and having nothing whatsoever to do with living patients. In reality the subject is much greater and has significant variety. The term 'pathology' is actually an umbrella heading for several subjects that are summarized below. As a generalization, the majority of the work will involve using specimens from the human body to help clinicians diagnose disease. This may include blood and other bodily fluids and also biopsy specimens. In this way the pathology services will be used by doctors from all fields – communication is thus essential. There is a dedicated exam for these specialties, the MRCPath. There will be opportunities for a small number of doctors to take posts in these specialties during their FY2 year but the majority will enter following the Foundation Programme and embark on run-through training, which will last for 5 years. The MRCPath is divided into two parts, which need to be completed at certain stages in order to continue.

Chemical pathology

This is otherwise known as biochemistry and involves the running of biochemical laboratories involved in the interpretation of investigation results. Doctors in this specialty also have clinic commitments where they manage and advise other clinicians about various metabolic disorders, for example patients with high cholesterol. It is also common for trainees to complete some research during their training.

Haematology

This specialty used to be laboratory-based but now the clinical component predominates. There is a significant inpatient and outpatient workload. Great variety can be seen with the conditions and one appealing factor is the complete management of the patient from the first abnormal blood test to diagnosis of the disorder, both clinically and by performing tests such as a bone marrow aspirate. The spectrum of disease ranges from abnormalities in the number of blood cells in the body, through clotting disorders and genetic problems, to haematological malignancies and blood transfusion conundrums. This specialty requires two sets of postgraduate exams to be passed: the MRCP during the first two ST years (core medical training years; see Chapter 20) and then the MRCPath during later training. Your workload as a consultant will depend on the type of hospital and area but it is possible to subspecialize in a specific area of haematology, for example bone marrow transplantation (some students find this term a little confusing – it should be noted that this does not require an operation and the transplant is supplied through a drip, in a similar way to a blood transfusion).

Histopathology/cytology

Histopathology involves the study of the function and structure of the tissue from a patient's body; cytology involves the study of the structure and function of cells. The examination of these tissues and cells using a microscope and special staining procedures can help to provide the diagnosis. As well as microscopic techniques, pathologists are also involved in performing autopsy examinations (dissection of a body to determine the cause of death). Research is common and, in the larger teaching hospitals, you can often develop an interest in one particular organ or system.

Microbiology

Here you will be involved in the management of clinical infections in both the hospital and the community. Much of the work will help clinicians in other specialties to isolate and determine microorganisms and to advise on appropriate treatment with antimicrobials (e.g. antibiotics). As well as being concerned about patient infections, part of the workload will involve education about the prevention of the spread of infection. Although it may seem from the outside that much of the time would be spent using a microscope, the work of the microbiologist involves clinical decision-making regarding difficult cases on the wards. There tends to be a particularly close relationship with doctors with an interest in infectious diseases. There are several subspecialties including virology and parasitology.

Ophthalmology

Ophthalmologists are concerned with treating diseases of the eye and visual system, from the contents of the orbit to the brain. Ophthalmology is considered to be somewhat of a hybrid of surgery and medicine – indeed there are many medical conditions that affect different parts of the body, such as disorders of the blood, heart and even joints, that are first apparent with symptoms related to the eye. The majority of patients are elderly, but usually not very unwell, and some require a long period of care, with many appointments in the outpatients department. Operations are usually short and conducted under local anaesthesia, and the surgery itself is usually very fine surgery, conducted under an operating microscope or with a laser, to treat diseases affecting the retina (the back of the eye). Ophthalmology, although considered to be a subspecialty of medicine and surgery, is now becoming further subdivided into the fields of corneal surgery (e.g. corneal transplantation), surgery of the orbit (e.g. orbital tumours), vitreoretinal surgery (treating such things as retinal detachments), paediatric ophthalmology and finally medical ophthalmology involving not surgery but treatment of diseases of the eye such as vascular and inflammatory disorders. The instruments particular to this specialty are the ophthalmoscope to peer into the eye, and the slit lamp which allows visualization of the lens and the back of the eye.

Training

Trainees will enter Ophthalmic Specialist Training (OST) following their Foundation Programme (some may have spent part of their FY2 year in the specialty but this will not be essential). The OST is a run-through training programme lasting 7 years and requires a trainee to complete the FRCOphth. The examination will be in two parts, with the first one having to be completed by the end of year 2. Failure to gain this will prevent progression. The second part is likely to be sat towards the end of year 4. As with all the specialties, trainees will have to demonstrate satisfactory progress in obtaining competencies in order to continue with their training.

Advantages
Combination of medicine and surgery, diagnosis often possible on examination alone, few emergencies so out-of-hours commitment less, long-term care of patients.

Disadvantages
Highly competitive, a lot of cataract operations.

Psychiatry

This involves studying and diagnosing mental illness as well as behavioural and emotional problems. It is a surprisingly large specialty, incorporating hospital as well as outpatient and community-based care. There is an emphasis on multidisciplinary team-working; doctors are only a small part of a large team of nurses and social workers and communication skills are essential. Most consultants will have a subspecialty interest (e.g. old age psychiatry, children and adolescents, substance misuse, forensic psychiatry). The postgraduate exam is the MRCPsych which will need to be completed during specialist training to allow progression. It involves a combination of multiple choice, essay, viva and clinical examinations. Compared with other specialties there tends to be less in the way of practical procedures and life on-call can be slightly more civilized.

Training
Foundation Programme followed by 6 years specialist training. Completion of the MRCPsych is required before application to ST3 posts.

Skills
Good at communicating, empathic.

Advantages
Flexible working, light on-call, interface with many other branches of medicine, good job opportunities, ability to work in large teams and in various locations.

Disadvantages
Chronic problems with the results of treatment often taking weeks to be seen, patients following through with their suicidal ideas, emotionally draining.

Radiology

Radiology doctors use X-rays and other imaging techniques to assist in disease diagnosis. As well as having an eye for detail required for interpreting these scans, some become interventional radiologists. This involves performing invasive procedures under scanning guidance, traditionally skills performed by physicians or surgeons. With the advance in imaging technology, it is now possible to become a consultant with a particular interest in one area, for example magnetic resonance imaging. Radiologists will investigate other consultant's patients and so communicating and liaising with the other teams is essential. This role is not to be mistaken with that of a radiographer who will actually perform many of the scans while the radiologist has the responsibility for interpreting the pictures. As well as a good knowledge of anatomy, a doctor in this specialty needs a good background in medical, surgical and pathological processes and their treatment. For this reason, although not compulsory, many trainees spend time in these specialties first, often gaining a diploma (e.g. MRCS). The actual Royal College of Radiologists diploma is the FRCR and this needs to be achieved to progress through to gain a CCT (Certificate of Completion of Training).

Training
Following the foundation years, radiology training is five run-through years and focuses on core skills in the first 3 years and then subspecialization in the final 2 years.

Skills
Good communication skills, fine eye for detail, dexterity for interventional procedures.

Advantages
Flexibility, rapidly advancing technology, reasonable on-call, expanding, autonomy (in control of your own scanners), well-structured training programme.

Disadvantages
Lack of follow-up of patients, can be seen as just a service specialty, extra exams.

Academic medicine

It is recognized that producing medically qualified academics is important for maintaining cutting edge clinical research and directing healthcare provision in the UK. However, over the last few decades the number of academic doctors has slowly declined. This was addressed in the Walport Report, which called for initiatives that integrated the development of academic skills with each of the key stages of a clinician's career. These academic pathways have now been created to attract doctors who have the potential to become leaders in clinical research and education.

The academic training pathway runs in parallel to the standard training and is available in most of the medical specialties (Figure 18.1). Academic FY1 and FY2 posts are available and these offer some dedicated time working with academic doctors to get a flavour for the work they do. Following

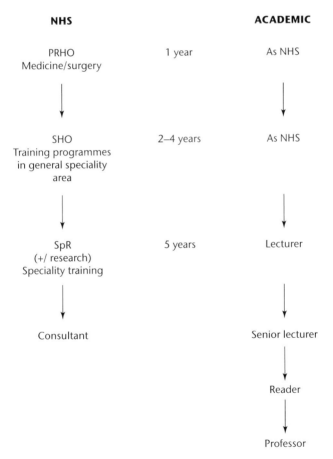

Figure 18.1 The academic training structure prior to MMC; see text for the description of the proposed new training structure

this there are competitive academic clinical fellowships (ACF), which are equivalent to core training posts. During this time, approximately 40% (2 days a week) of the trainee's time is spent in academic activity related to their specialty of interest. After this most trainees undertake full-time research for 2 or 3 years to obtain an MD or PhD before applying for a competitive clinical lectureship (CL) in their specialty. The CL post is usually split 50% research and 50% clinical activity. Following 6 or 7 years as a CL, the next steps are senior lecturer, followed by reader and then professor (each of these is equivalent to a consultant in clinical standing). Most academics will be jointly employed by the NHS and the university. Competition for posts is high and time management skills are essential to be able to balance the clinical commitments with research and teaching time. There is constant pressure to publish new results and obtain funding for running experiments or trials. The work is varied and enjoyable though.

Pharmaceutical industry

There are many doctors who decide that instead of treating patients directly, they would rather be involved in developing new drugs. Doctors work within all areas of the pharmaceutical industry: in laboratories with scientists discovering new drugs, running clinical trials where new drugs are tested on volunteers to see if they are safe and effective, with regulatory bodies that check that new drugs have gone through all the necessary tests, and in sales and marketing. The financial resources of the pharmaceutical industry can come as a (not unpleasant) shock after working in the cash-strapped NHS and the work can be exciting and intellectually stimulating. Many doctors miss patient contact; others see this as an advantage.

Most doctors enter the pharmaceutical industry after at least 3 years working as an NHS doctor, and postgraduate exams are becoming increasingly necessary. There are plans to introduce specialist registrar training in pharmaceutical medicine.

The armed services

It is possible to work as a doctor in one of the armed services. This choice can be made during university days and each medical school will normally hold a careers fair early in the third year. If a medical student decides at this point that he or she wishes to pursue this particular path, then the chosen armed force will sponsor the student through the clinical years (by covering tuition fees and paying an annual salary). In return you have to continue in employment for up to 6 years following graduation. If you leave before this time, then you would be responsible for paying some of the money back.

Many of the jobs offered by the armed forces will be based in the UK. The opportunities for travel will be easier and graduates could find themselves in countries at war. Spending time in the armed forces will not usually affect career progression but there may be some specialties in which it is difficult to obtain the correct exposure. Many of the early jobs will involve general practice-type duties. A further difference is that a few months may be spent doing general training with non-medical colleagues.

Non-medical

Despite 5 years at medical school, some people do decide that medicine is possibly not the vocation for them. Qualifying with a medical degree can open doors to a range of other non-medical jobs. Most doctors make the change some time after their first couple of years – this has given them enough experience to be sure and also allows them to achieve full registration in case of future need. Employers will look seriously at medical graduates because of their proven academic record and also the characteristics and skills they will have. On the downside they may question your dedication and staying power. Most of those leaving the hospital and GP circuit will seek careers not altogether foreign. These will include the pharmaceutical industry, medical journalism, medical law and holistic health opportunities. Outside of medicine altogether, the possibilities are endless. Some have moved to the bright lights of the capital city for careers in banking and finance, and one doctor in the Midlands even changed to driving a taxi. The reasons for changing career are usually personal. Pay and hours are poignant issues, but from the outside the grass can always appear greener, so be sure of your decision.

18.4 Summary

Until recently the number of doctors in this country was expanding at a rapid rate in order to cope with the reduction in hours governed by the European Working Time Directive. With the financial crisis in the NHS, this expansion has now been reduced and there is a real chance that doctors could find themselves unemployed. For this reason competition for places will increase and so it is essential to keep ahead of the game with regard to opportunities for improving your curriculum vitae. No other degree allows such variation in a graduate's ultimate job selection but it is essential to think carefully before choosing a particular specialty as it could become more difficult to change the further down the training path a doctor goes.

PERSONAL VIEW   *Adam Gordon*

It's Friday night. My children are in bed, the dishes are done and as my wife sits down to flick through the digibox, I take my leave and head off to a care home to carry on my day's research. I'd rather not be doing it but the Professor of Nursing would like to see data from me by the end of the month and I've been so busy, what with the teaching and the on-calls and the review articles I've been writing, that I need to push on.

It's been a funny sort of week, like a lot of my weeks. That comes from being a clinical academic, employed half the time by an acute NHS Trust and half by a university. Life is made even more varied by the fact I'm a community geriatrician, so over the course of a week I can be in a patient's front room working out why they're falling all the time, leading a resuscitation on a hospital ward, lecturing to undergraduates, presenting to an academic meeting and wading through research papers for a literature review.

On Monday, I was on-call for Medicine. I spent hours with a woman in the high-dependency unit who had multiorgan failure. I placed a central line and an arterial line, gave her broad-spectrum antibiotics and commenced her on inotropes. I told her family she probably wasn't going to make it. She didn't. They were expecting it, but it was difficult for them nevertheless. I sat with them for a while, talking. We discussed how she had got gradually less well over the preceding 12 months. She had started using a zimmer frame, become incontinent and gone into a care home. There she had fallen and broken her hip. After the operation she had a severe gastrointestinal bleed, probably because of the aspirin she was taking, was endoscoped and subsequently came to medical high dependency. There she developed a pneumonia. That had been on Monday morning, when I met her.

The rest of my week has been typically varied. One afternoon I taught student nurses about cognitive impairment (memory loss). I was allocated 3 hours. We discussed the term 'dementia' and what it means to both professionals and patients, we looked at CT scans, and we listened to a tape of Cliff Richard talking about how his mother died of dementia. At the end of the session, two nurses approached me. One told me how refreshing it was to have a doctor engage with them, to speak to them like equals and to teach them something new. The other one told me I was 'dishy'.

Over the course of the week I have spent hours wading through care home records, carefully recording details of residents' nutritional status, cognition, behaviour and functional dependency. It's arduous work; at times interesting, at times mind-numbingly repetitive. This is my research – trying to understand the medical needs of care home residents and to plot how these change over time. The aim is to be able to more effectively predict when residents will experience a decline, so that anticipatory care arrangements can be put in place. The reality, for the moment, is hours of wading through care home records, ticking boxes on preprinted forms.

Like most medical careers, it's a real mixed bag being an academic. There is glory, no doubt. It's a real buzz lecturing to a theatre full of students who are clearly enjoying your teaching, following what you say, learning from it. You can feel the love in a situation like that, especially if they think you're 'dishy'. Research, too, is rewarding. Imagine thinking of a research idea, nurturing it and chaperoning it through protocol writing, ethics applications and into the light of day. Then actually doing the research and, if it works, telling the medical profession something new about how to do its job. And then you write the article, see your name in print in a medical journal and a physician in another country, that you've never met, reads what you've written, reflects on what you've said, and changes their practice. That's pretty awesome – the fact that you can influence the care of patients you've never met.

It's also not without its downsides. There's juggling clinical and academic responsibilities. If you're phoned during an academic session about a sick patient, it can be difficult to say no. And there's the fact that academic work never goes away. When you leave a hospital after a clinical shift, work is finished for the day but, once you're home, your laptop is always there loaded with academic work, beckoning you to mark those essays, to spend just another few hours on that article. It takes a lot of discipline, sometimes, to switch off. There's the disappointment when you fall short of a deadline, when your work doesn't come up to scratch, your abstract rejected for a conference, your research article declined by a journal. Then there's all that extra training. I've been a competent doctor for a number of years, but I'm still a fledgling academic. In many ways, it's like starting over again. On the wards I'm the wise experienced veteran. In an academic meeting I'm often the wet-behind-the-ears rookie. Perhaps the biggest drain, though, is the sheer amount of effort required to do good research – the hours writing protocols, reading literature, gathering the same data from different people over and over again.

Back to the present. The missed opportunity of a rare night in front of the telly still in my mind, I arrive at the care home. I am greeted at the door by an old lady with dementia. She is distressed, trying to escape through the locked door. I talk to her calmly, listen to her complaints and, after five minutes or so, walk her back through the home to her room. She is grateful. I notice that she

(continued)

(*Continued*)

has a slightly parkinsonian gait and wonder if that's something to do with her medication. I return to the manager's office and sit down to wade through the notes some more.

It's at times like this, possibly, that it all comes together. What if I can learn enough about these residents' problems to influence the care of others like them. What if I can better understand the factors that lead to decline, that precipitate a catastrophe. How would this have influenced the life of the lady I saw in the high-dependency unit on Monday? What if we had found the cause for her failing mobility and she hadn't fallen and broken her hip at all. What if, when she had fallen, she had been managed palliatively in the care home. What if, when she had come to hospital, the limits of her care had been carefully discussed in advance, so that she had a calm controlled death in a side-room, instead of surrounded by monitors, with invasive lines in place, in the high-dependency unit.

I don't know the answer to these questions but I suspect that part of it might lie in the notes on the manager's desk in front of me. And this is how I make sense of my life as a clinical academic – my clinical work lets me make sense of my research, while my research lets me tackle head-on the big questions raised through my practice. That's the pay-off. I open the first set of notes and start ticking boxes – there's never anything on the telly anyway.

Chapter 19 **Training as a general practitioner**

Each general practitioner (GP) provides front-line care for about 2000 patients. GPs manage up to 90% of episodes of illness seen by all doctors, and as well as looking after chronic diseases they play a role in health promotion. Approximately 50% of doctors are GPs, although if you asked most first-year medical students whether they wanted to be GPs, the proportion would be much lower. The fact is most people start medical school at the age of 18 and do not know what area they want to specialize in. This is both normal and sensible because you do not know what the various jobs involve. Some people have a very strong idea about their chosen career, but it is surprising how many of these views will change with time.

Try to keep an open mind for as long as possible – there's no hurry! One point to remember is that at medical school the teaching in the clinical years is predominantly hospital-based. You may have a 4–6 week placement in general practice with one GP, but otherwise you are taught primarily by hospital physicians and surgeons. It is only natural while training to find people whom you admire and with whom you identify. It drives your ambition and influences your choice of career. However, you may meet over 100 hospital doctors compared with only one GP. This is obviously a little biased. Luckily things are changing and many medical schools now run teaching in the earlier years where students visit general practices on a regular basis.

General practice can offer a varied and interesting career with flexibility. Just don't forget it as an option.

19.1 The training requirements

The training for general practice is currently under review and is evolving. To become a GP takes a minimum of 5 years after graduating as a doctor.

The Essential Guide to Becoming a Doctor, 3rd edition. © Adrian Blundell,
Richard Harrison and Benjamin Turney. Published 2011 by Blackwell Publishing Ltd.

You will need to do your foundation training for 2 years and then complete three further years of specialist training. Currently, the training combines a number of 4-month posts in various hospital specialties as a specialty registrar (e.g. medicine, obstetrics and gynaecology, paediatrics, accident and emergency) and 20 months as a GP registrar (i.e. a training post within general practice; see later).

To do this you can join a vocational training scheme (VTS), which is a rotation of jobs specially designed for general practice. You apply for the scheme on a national basis and if successful on selection you are allocated jobs in the different specialties in a particular region. You often have some choice in the jobs you would like to do. You will also be allocated a job in general practice under the supervision of a GP trainer. One of the advantages of joining a VTS is that all your jobs are sorted out for you and you do not have to continually apply for new jobs every few months. This not only saves you hassle, but also gives you stability and allows you to live in one area. Other advantages of being part of a VTS include regular teaching, careers advice, information about exams and general support. It has previously been possible to arrange you own 'VTS scheme' independently; however, it is becoming increasingly difficult to do this and you should seek further advice before considering this option. You may also be able to include some experience gained working abroad if applicable, although you would need to check whether a particular job would be accredited for training by discussing this with the PMETB and local post organizers. All this training can be done part-time if you have a valid reason for doing so, such as having children.

Often many people entering general practice will have done more than the minimum requirement of jobs. You may start out training to be a paediatrician for example and later decide that it is not for you. Extra experience is seen as a positive attribute for being a GP; you will have additional specialist skills that can only be of benefit during your training and while practising as a GP. It is generally thought to be easier to change from a hospital career to general practice compared with the other way around, although this is still possible. As a general piece of advice, if you are unsure whether to be a GP or a hospital doctor, start with the hospital job and take things from there.

In addition, working overseas is also viewed in a positive light by GPs, although this will not influence your application. This is becoming more popular among all doctors, but has always been welcomed in general practice.

19.2 GP registrar

Being a GP registrar is a unique post. You will normally work as a GP registrar for 20 months. Depending on the VTS, this time is usually split between the hospital jobs, although a considerable proportion will be at the end.

The post usually involves a short period of introduction into the practice. This includes sitting in with GPs, practice nurses, midwives and going out visiting with the district nurses and health visitors. This gives you the opportunity to get to know the staff and find out exactly what everybody's job involves. You then start to see patients as if you were a GP, but usually with longer appointment times at first. You are, throughout, under the supervision of a GP trainer. These are GPs with a special interest in teaching and who have worked as a GP for at least 3 years. They will carry on doing their normal work, but you can ask them questions if necessary and they will give you regular teaching.

19.3 Imminent changes to GP training

In January 2008, Sir John Tooke's report on Modernizing Medical Careers recommended that training for general practice in the UK should be extended from 3 to 5 years, the report suggesting that this should be implemented by 2011. The first 'five-year' trainees will be those students currently in their final year at medical school, and they will therefore leave GP specialty training in 2016 at the earliest.

19.4 The exams

Changes introduced in 2008 mean that it is now compulsory to sit the Royal College of General Practitioners postgraduate membership exam (nMRCGP) to become an independent GP. The exam consists of three elements.

Applied Knowledge Test
A computer-based 3-hour multiple-choice test of 200 items, covering subjects such as clinical medicine, critical appraisal and evidence-based clinical practice, and health informatics and administrative issues.

Clinical Skills Assessment
A clinical exam in which you undertake 13 'mock' consultations, each of 10 minutes. Patients are played by trained role-players.

Workplace-based assessment
Essential evidence of competence, which is collected over all 3 years of training, recorded in a web-based e-portfolio, in essence similar to coursework from GCSE and A levels. Self-explanatory tools such as Multi-source Feedback, Patient Satisfaction Questionnaire and Direct Observation of Procedural Skills are among some of the tools used.

19.5 The image

I think it would be fair to say that general practice suffers from an image problem. You must have heard people referring to GPs as doctors wearing sandals and cardigans with leather elbow patches! I believe there are several reasons for this.

Many, but by no means all, hospital doctors develop a bad view of GPs. They feel they see unnecessary referrals to hospital, poor-quality referral letters and patients with missed diagnoses. These can all be frustrating while working in hospitals, especially when very busy, and I certainly remember indulging in some 'GP bashing' myself while working as a medical SHO. Now, there are some lower-quality GPs, just as there are poorer performing hospital doctors, but there are often legitimate reasons for missed diagnoses and unnecessary referrals. The lung cancer in a smoker may be quite obvious by the time he or she presents to hospital with 2-stone weight loss, coughing blood and an abnormality on the chest X-ray, but may not have been so when the GP saw the patient 3 months ago with 'a bit of a tickly cough'. Equally, it can be frustrating that an old lady who fell at home and has broken her wrist has to be admitted to hospital, but if she cannot get to the toilet because she cannot get out of her chair and she has no friends or family to help her then there may be nowhere else for her to go. These things are hardly the fault of GPs, but we are easy to blame.

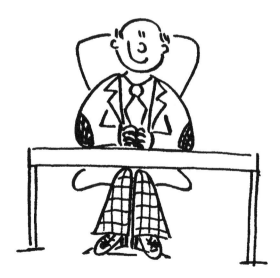

I think it would be fair to say that general practice suffers from an image problem

I believe that the introduction of general practice into many foundation schemes will help to change this. Hopefully now a large number of doctors will gain some first-hand experience of working in general practice and the challenges that it raises. This may also help with another common misconception that general practice is boring. A lot of my contemporaries truly seem to believe this. You hear comments such as 'I couldn't cope with seeing all those coughs and colds' or 'Don't you get tired of seeing earache?' Boring is one thing that general practice is not. Certainly there are routine parts to it like any hospital specialty, but the truth is you never know what will come through the door next. It might be someone who has just found out she is pregnant, someone whose wife died yesterday, someone with his or her first presentation of a brain tumour, or someone having a heart attack. Obviously if you work in hospital and perceive general practice as boring, you may also regard those doctors who choose it as inferior. Certainly when I first decided to be a GP I was very careful about whom I told – 'It's a waste' and 'You'll be so bored' were common comments. I do not want to cast all hospital doctors in this light. Many actually admire GPs and go out of their way to be helpful during hospital SHO training posts and later in teaching GPs. Also I do not believe general practice is for everyone (see later), but the point I am making is that general practice often gets a bad press in hospitals, and as that is where you spend a great deal of time as a student and junior doctor, some of it no doubt rubs off.

Finally, there has been a lot of coverage in the media recently about low morale in general practice and the lack of GPs. In fact there is usually some medical story in the news each week and this applies equally to hospital medicine – bed shortages, waiting lists, and so on. It is important not to become disillusioned and form your own opinions. However, there are other more subtle media influences. On an evening spent at home, if you had a choice would you rather watch *ER* or *Doctors*? Not a tricky decision really! Give me the excitement and good looks of those glossy hospital dramas any day. I am not even going to try to pretend that being a GP is as exciting as an episode of *ER*, thank goodness, but then most A&E jobs are not either. The general public do not think that general practice is as sexy as being a brain surgeon, but you probably realize that.

19.6 Working as a GP

Being a GP is about being a generalist as opposed to a specialist. This may seem obvious but is an important point. A colleague once described general practice as 'specializing in being a generalist'. You are expected to know a little bit about a lot, rather than a lot about a little. This certainly does not appeal to everyone. You will never be a complete authority on a subject. In fact you will end up with a very good knowledge of some of the common general practice problems, but you need to realize your limitations and be prepared to refer to a specialist if necessary. Increasingly, GPs are being encouraged to develop areas of special interest, but you would still be expected to continue with your usual surgeries in addition. With a special interest it is possible to spend some sessions working in the local hospitals under the guidance of a consultant, for example in A&E.

There are other important aspects about general practice that differ from working in hospitals. As a GP you are self-employed rather than being employed by a hospital. This means that you have more influence over your working conditions, hours and pay. It also means more involvement in managerial and financial skills. In the current political climate, general practice, along with the rest of the NHS, is constantly evolving. In the recent past, the way in which GPs are paid has been reformed by a new contract that encourages GPs to meet targets called Quality Outcome Framework (QOF) points. GPs are currently joining together in groups that will be able to buy in services from hospitals in a scheme called practice-based commissioning. There are constantly new challenges to face in the structure and organization of general practice. This aspect of general practice appeals to some and can have its advantages in the sense of autonomy, but importantly there are an increasing number of jobs that do not require you to become as involved in these aspects if they do not appeal to you.

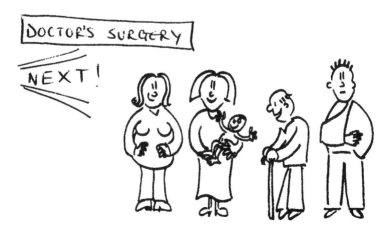

General practice can offer a varied and interesting career

General practices vary enormously and there is no such thing as a typical practice. You can work alone as a single-handed GP or in a large practice with many other partners. You can choose to work in the inner city or in a very rural area. As GPs are self-employed, it means that they can opt to do things in many different ways. This refers more to the organization of the practice than the medical decisions. For example, there are some GP practices around the country where GPs help run small so-called community hospitals. Here they can supervise the care of their own patients in hospital, help run minor injuries units (like a scaled-down A&E) and even help out on the maternity wards or other specialist areas. They can have direct access to X-ray facilities and sometimes do their own minor operations.

Thus one of the main advantages of general practice is the flexibility. This can often appeal to women who are thinking of having children, but may also appeal if you have other interests both medical and non-medical. As a full-time GP you will usually work eight or nine sessions per week (a session is a morning or afternoon surgery plus paperwork), which means one or two half days off per week. It is common to find jobs that are three-quarter time, usually six to seven sessions per week, or part-time (four to five sessions per week). Most practices will do their own on-call during the day but in the evenings and weekends most will now use a cooperative or deputizing service. Essentially, large numbers of practices join together to provide an on-call service. You may be required to do the on-call, but this usually only works out at around two to three sessions per month. Basically, general practice often appeals to people who want a life outside of medicine or increased variety in their work. This is obviously possible with a career in a hospital specialty, but it is usually harder. However, be under no illusion, being a GP is hard work and is not an easy option, and general practice is often described as a lifestyle choice.

Finally, it is important to consider the other aspects involved in general practice. Communication skills are very important. You need to work as part of a team with other health professionals (e.g. other GPs, practice nurses and health visitors), and remember that some of them will be your employees. All doctors need to be able to communicate effectively with patients, but especially in general practice where you will look after your patients for many years. This may not always be an advantage if the patient is difficult, but mostly it offers a unique opportunity for you to build relationships with patients and their families. You also have the opportunity to see patients in their own environment, which is very different to talking to someone in a hospital bed. It allows you develop understanding of how illness can have an effect on a person's daily life, including home, work and relationships.

19.7 Summary

If you had asked me at the start of medical school whether I wanted to be a GP, I would have said no. If you were to ask me whether I am happy with my career choice now, I would say yes. General practice is challenging, flexible and fun and I can see myself doing it for the rest of my career. Don't rule it out.

PERSONAL VIEW   *James Hopkinson*

I trained at Nottingham Medical School and had a fantastic time as a student. I knew exactly what my career path was going to be; I was going to be an orthopaedic surgeon, a trauma specialist. I was particularly dismissive of general practice – I didn't want to be a 'second-rate' doctor!

Things changed when my house jobs started, and I realized how little time would be spent doing 'exciting' trauma cases and how much time would be spent doing 'boring' ward rounds and paperwork. I also realized that when the trauma usually happened I would prefer to be asleep! With some trepidation I began exploring other possibilities. I spent some time with GPs and saw that they were in control of what they did, and when they did it. I saw the opportunities to get involved in areas of medicine that interested them, as opposed to the hospital doctors who appeared to have little freedom in their working practices.

I joined the Nottingham VTS straight from house jobs and never looked back. The general practice training was split into two 6-month posts at the beginning and the end of my 3-year rotation. In between consisted of 6 months each of psychiatry, general medicine, obstetrics and gynaecology, and paediatrics. The MRCGP exam followed my final 6 months and then I decided to take advantage of the flexibility general practice allows, and did a 6-month post in sports and exercise medicine, a new and unique post. This was funded by the postgraduate dean as part of an ongoing programme to create GPs with special interests (GPSIs). I gained my diploma in sports medicine, and decided that I wanted to continue to work within sports medicine. Almost concurrently a partnership in a local village became available. I was hesitant to begin with as there are so many opportunities to locum, which carry no long-term commitment. The practice was very well set up, was forward thinking, and most of all I liked the people there. I subsequently applied and was offered the job. During discussion with the other partners I emphasized my desire to continue to work within sports medicine and they were all supportive and flexible.

My initial contract was for 6 months. I found I very much enjoyed the working environment, but I had a steep learning curve ahead of me. Suddenly I had more responsibilities than just the medical care of my patients. I was now self-employed, running my own business. The practice employs 35 staff – people management is not part of medical training. Fortunately, the other partners were very helpful during my settling-in period and made time to help me out. I also found the paperwork mountain that I had been told about but never really believed. It is true that when you become a partner the floodgates open!

As the practice owned its own buildings, this meant 'buying' into the practice. This involved taking out a mortgage that was bigger than my house mortgage, to buy out the preceding partner. Fortunately, the PCT pay rent on the premises, which at present interest rates more than covers the cost of the mortgage. This will hopefully create a nice tax-free lump sum when I retire, and the next person buys in.

Within 6 months I was approached by a professional Olympic team that trains locally asking if I would be interested in looking after them medically. I was obviously very interested, but a little scared as I had never looked after an amateur side. I agreed to do it jointly with a well-established sports doctor in the area, while I gained more experience. Since then I have travelled with several British teams around the world. I have been medical officer to the World University Games in Korea and Turkey, and I was also involved in the Winter Olympics in Turin. General practice allows me the flexibility to earn a good salary while pursuing my special interest.

I love my job, and I would not change it for the world.

Chapter 20 **Training in the medical field (becoming a physician)**

To talk about a career in a medical specialty, it is helpful to first define the term 'general medicine'. It can certainly cause some confusion because at university the course is called medicine, but a career in a medical specialty is different. General medicine is a term that has been used historically. It can also be referred to as internal medicine and involves the diagnosis and treatment of diseases of the internal organs. In simple terms it could be thought of as all the specialties excluding surgery, general practice, anaesthetics, radiology and laboratory sciences. Traditionally, this definition was close to the truth. However, in the modern age there has been diversion of many specialties away from general medicine, a good example being paediatrics. The subspecialization has come about as technology and medicine become more complex and so a consultant needs to be very knowledgeable in one particular area. General medicine still exists and will continue to do so. More recently, a specialty of acute medicine has been introduced. The training in many of the specialties within medicine will lead to dual accreditation. Roughly translated, this means a consultant physician is a specialist in one area but also takes part in the unselected general medical admission process. Not all subspecialties in medicine have general medical commitments, but this will depend on the individual hospital.

20.1 The hospital structure

The medical department in a hospital is divided into specialties, which in turn are divided into medical firms. These consist of a consultant, specialty registrars and foundation doctors. Not all firms will have the same number at each grade. The majority of the work for the more junior members of the team is to look after the general day-to-day activities on the ward. This will

The Essential Guide to Becoming a Doctor, 3rd edition. © Adrian Blundell,
Richard Harrison and Benjamin Turney. Published 2011 by Blackwell Publishing Ltd.

include a daily review of each patient and organizing and chasing the results of tests. The more senior registrars and consultants will have more clinic and procedure commitments depending on the specialty.

Common medical specialties

- Acute medicine
- Cardiology*
- Clinical oncology*
- Clinical pharmacology*
- Dermatology*
- Endocrinology
- Gastroenterology
- Genitourinary medicine*
- Haematology*
- Healthcare of the elderly
- Infectious diseases
- Medical oncology*
- Nephrology*
- Neurology*
- Palliative medicine*
- Rehabilitation*
- Respiratory medicine
- Rheumatology*

* Not always involved in general medicine

20.2 General medicine

Each day there will be a team of doctors in each hospital, under the guidance of a consultant, allocated to admitting patients. This means that all new patients referred to the hospital with medical conditions will come under the care of this consultant. Patients can be referred by the general practitioner or casualty, or be admitted following a 999 emergency ambulance call. These patients tend to be seen initially by the junior doctors, who will perform a medical history (ask some relevant questions) and an appropriate examination, and commence treatment as required. Following the history and examination, it is usual to determine a differential diagnosis, i.e. several possible explanations for the patient's symptoms. The patients will be reviewed by senior colleagues on a post-take ward round. Following review on this central admissions ward, the patients can then be moved to other wards depending on their medical needs and also their diagnosis, or discharged home if appropriate. Other information regarding on-call can be found in Chapters 15–17.

Examples of medical complaints seen by general physicians

- Chest pain
- Shortness of breath
- Chronic bronchitis
- Stroke
- Infections
- Blood clots
- Diabetes
- Bowel problems
- Confusion

20.3 Foundation years

Several posts during the Foundation Programme will be in medical specialties. The majority of a trainee's time will be spent looking after the patients on the ward. Each patient needs to be seen daily, with the senior doctors doing two or three rounds a week. Your role is important as you have the most contact with the patients, relatives and other healthcare professionals. A good foundation doctor will have excellent knowledge of their patients, including up-to-date information of the medical problems, results of tests, investigations pending and their social history. It is important to keep good medical records and know when to ask for advice and assistance. When on-call, it may be necessary to leave the team ward and spend the day or night on the admissions ward. There will be other members of the team to cover the consultant's patients on these occasions. During the Foundation Programme it is necessary to show adequate completion of the competencies expected as outlined in the training portfolio. Each doctor will be allocated an educational supervisor who will organize meetings throughout the year to check on progress. Many of the patients will require practical procedures to be carried out (see box below). These vary in complexity and as a doctor progresses up the training ladder, they should acquire experience starting with the simple ones first.

20.4 Specialist training (Basic Medical Training, i.e. ST1 and ST2)

The training grades SHO and SpR have been replaced with the specialty training registrar (StR). These changes were introduced in August 2007.

Chapter 15 outlines the new generic training ladder (see Figure 15.2). Following the Foundation Programme a doctor interested in pursuing a career in a physician specialty will need to apply for specialist training. The first 2 years of this will be known as Basic Medical Training (BMT), and following successful completion of this a trainee can continue to Higher Specialty Training (HST). There are two BMT programmes that a successful foundation doctor can apply for in order to continue to become a physician: Core Medical Training (CMT) and Acute Care Common Stem (ACCS). The majority of trainees will enter the CMT pathway. ACCS is a stem shared with anaesthetics and emergency medicine and so a trainee could follow one of these paths as an alternative or continue HST in medicine. Like the Foundation Programme, each component of the training will require adequate demonstration of competencies.

Each of the years will be divided into various 4- to 6-month placements. During CMT a trainee will rotate through different medical specialties in order to increase knowledge and experience.

During the first two CMT years, a trainee physician will still spend a large part of the time looking after the ward patients. As seniority develops other opportunities will arise, such as seeing patients in the outpatient department and performing specialist procedures, for example a training respiratory physician will spend time developing skills in bronchoscopy (a bronchoscope is a camera that looks into the lungs). Communication remains, as ever, an essential part of the job: patients (and relatives) require up-to-date knowledge of their conditions and you need to liaise with other healthcare professionals and specialists when organizing investigations. To continue in medical training, part of the competencies will be to pass the physician postgraduate examination, the diploma of the Royal College of Physicians, which allows you to become a Member of the Royal College of Physicians (MRCP). Obtaining the MRCP (UK) Diploma does not mean you have gained specialist status but this qualification is required for entry to HST.

Practical procedures in general medicine

- *Phlebotomy*: taking blood samples
- *Insertion of cannula*: small tube inserted into a vein to allow the administration of drugs and fluids
- *Arterial blood gases*: puncturing the radial artery to obtain a blood sample to measure the level of oxygen
- *Bladder catheterization*: insertion of a tube into the bladder to allow drainage of urine

(continued)

(*Continued*)

- *Central (venous) line*: insertion of a tube into a large vein, for example jugular vein, for administration of fluids
- *Lumbar puncture*: small needle used to obtain specimens of cerebrospinal fluid from the spinal cord
- *Needle aspiration*: needle inserted into a body cavity to obtain specimen of fluid
- *Drain insertion*: tube inserted into body cavity to drain fluid

20.5 Specialist training (Higher Specialty Training)

After completion of CMT or equivalent, a doctor will need to apply for (competitive) entry into the subspecialty of their choice. The initial part of specialty training will be broad-based training and, as a doctor progresses, the work will become more limited to the actual chosen specialty. As a more senior doctor (i.e. the equivalent of the current SpR grade), your seniority should in general reflect your clinical responsibilities. As well as outpatient and specialist procedure experience, you will be required to see patients with specialty problems under different hospital teams and advise on their management (e.g. surgical patients who have developed a medical problem). You will also be responsible for reviewing patients who become unwell or those who your juniors are concerned about. Other aspects of your work will include more managerial roles and taking part in audit, research and teaching. During this time it will also be possible (and in some specialties compulsory) to undertake a period of formal research (e.g. PhD). This will mean 2–3 years outside clinical medicine and on-calls, which could improve quality of life but can lead to a big reduction in pay (see Chapter 12 for more information about research). As already mentioned, not all medical specialties are involved in general medicine and some actually require further examinations to be taken during HST (e.g. clinical oncology and haematology). One other point to mention is that although the MRCP has been taken and the medical rotation completed, some doctors do not remain in the medical field and transfer to other specialties, such as general practice, radiology or A&E, where the MRCP is a useful but not an essential qualification.

During HST a doctor should gain the clinical specialist knowledge required to become a hospital consultant. It is also necessary to take an interest in audit, research and managerial aspects. Providing that training has been satisfactory, with completion of the assessments and core competencies as recorded in the training portfolios, the end of the programme leads to a Certificate of Completion of Training (CCT, previously known as CCST). This means that a doctor has his or her name on the specialist register and can be an independent practitioner. This qualification is recognized throughout Europe.

20.6 Member of the Royal College of Physicians Diploma

This postgraduate exam has undergone major changes over the last 5 years. It is divided into two parts with three distinct components (Part 1 written, Part 2 written and Part 2 clinical). Part 1 is divided into two papers with 100 questions each. These are in the 'best of five' format and will test knowledge of common disorders in general medicine and clinical sciences. Recent changes mean that the exam is criterion-referenced and negative marking has been abolished. Criterion referencing means an external assessment is made and a pass mark set rather than the old system of norm-referencing where a certain percentage of candidates were allowed to pass. The Part 2 written exam consists of three papers of around 100 questions. The format is a combination of 'best of five' and 'n from many' (choose several answers from a list). The questions will involve clinical scenarios and test a candidate's knowledge of diagnosis, investigation, management and prognosis. In this way the Part 2 written tends to be more relevant to the daily work of a trainee. The Part 2 clinical exam is called PACES (Practical Assessment of Clinical Examination Skills) and consists of five stations. This type of examination format is similar to the OSCE (Objective Structured Clinical Examination) that most medical schools now use for examining students. Each of the following systems is tested from a clinical perspective: cardiovascular, respiratory, abdominal, nervous and musculoskeletal (including eyes, skin and endocrine). To emphasize the importance of communication skills, two stations test this modality.

These exams require a significant amount of studying, which can prove difficult during a busy clinical job. Doctors are entitled to study leave and most hospitals provide a protected half day of teaching each week for their trainees. The other downside to having to sit the exam is the cost. There may be some money available for trainees to attend study courses but most of the examination fees have to be met personally. The total cost for the MRCP in 2010 is just over £1300 and that is if you are successful in passing all parts first time.

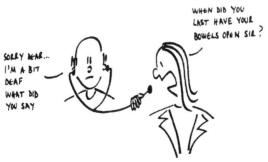

Training in the medical field

20.7 The consultant

After HST it is possible to apply for a hospital consultant post in your chosen specialty. At each step during your training there will be fewer jobs available and hence more competition. To ensure a top teaching hospital job, you often need a further qualification in the form of an MD or PhD. The work of consultants will involve more management and administration than that of their juniors. In total it could take up to 15 years from graduation before taking up a consultant post. Although, once a consultant, you have reached the top of the career ladder, it is still essential that you remain up to date, especially with the introduction of revalidation (see Chapter 17). Continuing medical education (CME) will ensure that consultants keep up to date with the latest developments and treatments. In order to continue practising medicine, you must collect a certain amount of CME points each year. These can be gained from various sources, but usually by attending educational seminars and courses. Most trainees find the transition to being a consultant stressful as the responsibility of the patient now lies with the most senior person, i.e. you. Many also find the amount of paperwork associated with being a consultant much greater than they could imagine. In this litigious society, other stressful times can involve being called to a coroner's court. Another major role is that of training and teaching medical students, junior doctors and other healthcare professionals. On the plus side, you are now a specialist in your own right and this will in general mean working less antisocial hours (depending on your specialty) and it is certainly possible to be invited as a guest speaker to various conferences both locally and internationally. Once an independent practitioner it is also possible to set up a private practice. The size and opportunity for this will depend a great deal on personal preference and specialty.

20.8 A day in the life

The weekly timetable for any consultant, including consultant physicians, is split into sessions. Each session within the normal working week is 4 hours and is known as a PA (programmed activity). Most consultant contracts are for 10 PAs, although this can be increased when 'outside' normal working hours is taken into consideration. Not all sessions are for direct clinical care as consultants need to be involved in management, teaching and also keeping themselves up to date. The normal working day is 9 a.m. to 5 p.m., although it is rare for the work to remain within these hours. On average a physician would spend two sessions doing a ward round of the patients under his or her care in the hospital, two sessions seeing patients in an outpatient clinic, one to two sessions performing a practical skill (e.g. endoscopy), one session for administration, one session for teaching, one session for CME and one session of on-call commitments. This timetable will vary considerably depending on the specialty as will the out-of-hours commitment. Most consultants would have several educational or multidisciplinary meetings each week, usually during lunch hours.

20.9 Summary

Training to be a physician is hard work but extremely rewarding. CMT is an essential grounding for all future physicians and can lead to a wide variety of possible subspecialties, which can vary from hospital to community and practical to non-practical.

PERSONAL VIEW   *Jeremy Snape*

I qualified in 1974 from Birmingham University after a largely undistinguished undergraduate 5 years. Not that my subsequent career has been any more feted. It has been rather makeshift and piecemeal in fact, at least until I settled on geriatric medicine. Nevertheless, it has been varied and interesting and I have enjoyed it.

As an undergraduate, I had no idea what I wanted to do and was late with my house-job applications and ended up in Shrewsbury (medicine) and Worcester (surgery). Fortuitous really, as both were lovely towns surrounded by idyllic countryside and also there was at least one decent boss in each place (Peter Boardman and Paul Smart). During that year I decided that I would like to work in Africa, although I was unprepared and knew relatively little about Third World medicine. To that end I applied for and got an SHO year in paediatrics in Carshalton, and from that was appointed as Medical Officer for Save the Children Fund (SCF) in Upper Volta, an ex-French colony in West Africa. The job started in October 1976, the year of the long hot summer. The focus was on prevention and management of endemic diseases and malnutrition. We, a team comprising nurses, health visitor, mechanic, local animateurs, a field director and myself, were based in a large village in the north (Gorom Gorom) surrounded by many smaller settlements. At base there was a small health centre with a clinic, pharmacy, laboratory and a six-bed ward where some more acute problems were dealt with. The bulk of the job, however, involved the mobile team (*équipe mobile*) visiting outlying villages each month. Talks and demonstrations were offered on how to avoid diarrhoea, parasites, malnutrition, malaria and measles among other problems.

(continued)

(*Continued*)

These sessions were led by our most charismatic animateur, Abdoulaye. This was a relatively innocent time in Africa, pre HIV/AIDS, pre internet and mobile phones, and before tarmac roads. I remained in Upper Volta for 2 years, and halfway through took 3 months out to study for the Diploma of Tropical Medicine and Hygiene in Liverpool. An excellent, stimulating and sociable experience.

Towards the end of 1979 ('winter of discontent'), I was starting to feel uneasy about the future, rather isolated and unsure of my future direction, and also feeling rusty in terms of medical skills and knowledge. So I returned to UK with the goal of obtaining the MRCP and then possibly to look for a post in general practice (the rural idyll). Sunderland General was a busy district general hospital, a good place to work for the first part of the MRCP; a good place to meet your future wife. I passed that part of the exam on the second attempt, in the nick of time, as it allowed me to get onto a registrar rotation in Liverpool where, after 2 years and three attempts, I nailed Part 2 of the diploma. The rural idyll in 1983 turned out to be disappointing. I found general practice claustrophobic and not for me, and after 9 months left to take up a registrar post in geriatric medicine back in Liverpool. The reasons for choosing geriatrics were pragmatic: it seemed more likely that I would get a job after my messy career path and it also seemed, demographically, that it was a specialty with a secure future. Of course it was a 'Cinderella' discipline – doctors in other medical subspecialties were somewhat sniffy about it. This in itself was a good reason to join its ranks.

The choice has been fortunate and although I made heavy weather of progressing to my consultant post (1988, Mansfield), it has been worth it. I worked for some inspirational characters during my training (Ray Tallis in Liverpool and Mark Castleden in Leicester the latter training me in the assessment and management of incontinence). Also in Leicester, Tony Wicks taught me endoscopy, which has been the precursor to an interest in nutrition.

On starting in Mansfield, there were two colleagues in geriatric medicine. They were isolated from the rest of the medical division, being based in the old Victorian workhouse, carrying out some multidisciplinary rehabilitation of patients transferred from two local district general hospitals. They were doing more than 300 domiciliary visits per year and participating in no acute unselected take and no postgraduate activities. Gradually, there was a coming together of our department with the rest of the medical division – we joined the on-take rota, a weekly medical clinical meeting was started and also a weekly multidisciplinary geriatrics meeting was launched. On appointment

I was given a weekly session for endoscopy, which was useful for our department as it allowed colleagues to get gastrointestinal investigations done easily and quickly. The gastroenterologist (Gordon Birnie) taught me to insert percutaneous endoscopic gastrostomy (PEG) tubes in the early 1990s. These tubes have become increasingly centre stage as nutrition has become an issue in many clinical situations: stroke, chronic neurological disease including dementia, and head and neck cancer. The ethical aspect of nutrition in frail and vulnerable patients has become a preoccupation and with the formation of the nutrition board and enteral nutrition group in 2003, we have had a proper forum to air concerns.

My other special interest is incontinence, the 'silent epidemic'. Again the hospital has been supportive. Soon after appointment, with a urologist (John Lemberger) and a gynaecologist (Clive Pickles) I put together the Continence Roadshow which visited 20 general practices in the area to discuss incontinence in all its aspects. I opened the continence centre with urodynamic equipment provided by the Trust. A continence nurse adviser was already in post and over time two more have been recruited.

From the early 1990s, I got involved in management, first as a clinical tutor, then as chair of the medical division and subsequently as Associate Director for Geriatric Medicine. In these roles I was part of teams which opened the new education centre, oversaw changes in medical training and guided the evolution of the medical take. I am still involved in management to some extent, having responsibility for registrars in geriatric medicine. Teaching too has been increasingly an area of endeavour. Undergraduates started coming to Kings Mill Hospital in the early 1990s. I enjoy teaching. In the late 1990s I became an examiner for the MRCP. We have hosted the exam four times at Kings Mill Hospital. I had a gap and had to retrain but this year I have started to examine again.

Geriatrics is a great specialty. Multidisciplinary working is often cited as one of the reasons for choosing the specialty. Individuals have varying levels of skill and energy (as in all professions), but when I have worked with dedicated physiotherapists, occupational therapists and social workers, it has been one of the joys. Admiring their expertise, working together towards a common goal, engaging in banter. In the gym the other day, I was seeing some patients with the physiotherapist. An older woman said to the physiotherapist, within my hearing, 'He's a nice doctor, if only I was 20 years younger and he wasn't married.' 'Yes', said the physio, 'If I had a pound for the number of times I've heard that, then I'd have two pounds!'

(*continued*)

(*Continued*)

Clinical geriatrics is unceasingly interesting, complex and challenging. Not only the variety and multiplicity of pathology and clinical conditions, but also the judgement required to be fair, kind and logical/honest with patients: to investigate and treat where appropriate and to accept when someone is approaching the end of life (i.e. dying). There has been a dearth of literature about disease in old age, although this is changing. Nevertheless, there are still plenty of opportunities to write about your patients: research, reviews, case reports. This is something I have done and I recommend it as a way of capturing ideas and patients. All too often we lose thoughts, moments, successes, failures. Getting them down in writing or print is a way of nailing them, stopping them from escaping. Slowing things down.

Perhaps the best thing about geriatric medicine is the patients as people. Of course there is a spectrum and I do not want to be over-sentimental; we do have our heart-sinking and revolving-door patients like all specialties. Perhaps it relates to their life experience – living through the Second World War, working as colliers, bringing up large families, seeing the mines close – I don't know, but they seem solid people of some depth, interested in life. Maybe I could share some stories.

Female 76, continence clinic, 6 months of failing memory. Her husband told me that during the miners' strike Arthur Scargill and Bruce Kent came to talk to the miners. On both occasions the chairperson did not turn up and twice his wife stood in, made the introductions, coordinated the questions and gave the vote of thanks. He was proud of her.

Female 92, outpatients. She had blood tests suggestive of Addison's disease and had been invited back for another test to exclude this diagnosis. When told this she said 'Jane Austen died of Addison's disease at 40. I'm 92 and as fit as a fiddle. I will not be your guinea-pig. Do you know the works of Jane Austen?' I say that I have read *Pride and Prejudice*. She says '*Sense and Sensibility* is better, perhaps the best.' I say I have seen the film. 'Ah yes', says she, 'Emma Thompson. Very faithful to the book, actually.' She went off agreeing to return if she felt unwell.

It is not uncommon to meet women in their eighties with a taste for bawdy humour.

Female 88, continence clinic. Shared a joke. Little boy asks his mum 'What's a penis?' 'That thing hanging between your dad's legs is a penis.' A little later he asks 'What's a twat?' 'Well', says his mum, 'that's the rest of him.'

Is geriatric medicine still a cinderella specialty? Well, it will never be glamorous like some, but while we are at the heart of things, participating in the on-call and in postgraduate activities and teaching, helping colleagues with complex patients by advising or taking them over, people are slowly realizing the contribution we make. Pursuing special interests may also contribute to the sum of knowledge. Doctors in other specialties are no longer as disparaging as they were 20 years ago.

I would not presume to offer advice to anyone unless they sought it. However, some thoughts might include the following.

- Be competent, be thorough, be nice to patients (and relatives).
- Develop a special interest; it's good to have one's own area of expertise.
- Ask unscripted questions: it may allow you to find out what makes your patient tick. They can be full of surprises.
- Write it down, keep a diary, publish, otherwise you will forget, lose precious episodes.
- Read: books about medicine and doctors, novels, observational literature, biography. Books about old age and ageing. Books about Africa. It will broaden horizons.

Postscript

This year, I participated in a 4-week course in Blantyre, Malawi entitled Tropical Medicine in Practice (the Trust were very accommodating). It was an excellent experience, completed as a refresher with a view to doing some voluntary work/teaching in Africa after retirement in a year or two.

Chapter 21 **Training in the surgical field**

The dictionary definition of surgery is '[that] branch of medicine that treats diseases, injuries, and deformities by manual or operative methods' – in other words, using physical intervention as a cure. Surgery can be a very satisfying profession, with a mixture of analytical and manual skills. There can be disadvantages, mainly long hours and commitments that often interfere with your personal life, but all the effort can be worthwhile. As most surgeons will tell you, there is no specialty like surgery, where you can have fun as well as get the chance to perform life-saving and life-improving operations.

21.1 History of surgery

Surgery has been performed since prehistoric times, when sharpened flints and other sharp-edged devices were used to perform such surgical operations as circumcision. The early Greeks and Romans practised surgery with great skill and with such cleanliness that infection of surgical and other wounds was relatively uncommon. During the Middle Ages surgical practice fell into the hands of the unskilled and uneducated. The barber-surgeon, who performed the usual functions of a barber as well as surgical operations, became a common figure, especially in Britain and France. It was not until the 18th century that surgery began to reach a professional level. With the introduction of antiseptic methods, surgery entered its modern phase. Louis Pasteur established the fact that microbes are responsible for infection and disease, and Joseph Lister was the first to discover the principles of antisepsis (the prevention of the spread of infection), prior to which about 80% of surgical patients contracted gangrene. In the 19th century, anaesthesia was developed and radically changed surgical practice. In the 20th century,

The Essential Guide to Becoming a Doctor, 3rd edition. © Adrian Blundell,
Richard Harrison and Benjamin Turney. Published 2011 by Blackwell Publishing Ltd.

the development of surgical instruments revolutionized the practice, and the introduction of modern imaging techniques and technology, such as the heart–lung bypass machine, have made the impossible possible, for example heart transplantation and tumour excision.

21.2 The career

As with any career, you should think about what you are good at and what you are looking for in your future job. The general attributes of a good surgeon include the following.

- Making decisions: can you think on your feet and learn from mistakes?
- Lifelong learning: would you like to have a career where you need to constantly update your knowledge?
- Building up trust: could you explain things clearly to patients and other doctors in your team?
- Manual dexterity and spatial awareness.

The first three are attributes for doctors in most specialties, but one of the big differences in surgery is the addition of the fourth. If you prefer working alone, hate learning new things and crack under pressure, surgery may not be for you. However, surgery can be an extremely enjoyable, intellectually demanding and satisfying career.

Surgeons have traditionally been stereotyped as having certain personalities. One opinion is that they should be male, athletic, possessed of a vocabulary of single syllables, have the endurance of a marathon runner, and maintain a political, social and sexual orientation somewhere to the right of Attila the Hun. Is this stereotype fair? Some surgeons may fit the bill, but in general this description is unfair. It is hoped that the methods and manner of characters such as Sir Lancelot from the film *Doctor in the House* are disappearing. The other main fault with the above description can be seen if the number of women now entering surgery is taken into account.

Other changes have come about with the introduction of the Patients' Charter. Surgeons are no longer considered as god-like people who can do only good. It is necessary for them to communicate well and explain why a patient needs the operation they are offering. With the advent of the internet, patients are much more knowledgeable. Although a considerable amount of time will be spent in the operating theatre, a surgeon will have many other commitments. Those consultants with an interest in surgical research can choose to work in academic units. Consultants can also opt to have contracts with NHS trusts so that they can continue to work in both clinical practice and research. Those with academic intentions can be appointed as lecturers, senior lecturers or readers, perhaps leading subsequently to a chair (position of professor) in surgery. Other consultants spend some of their time in private practice and surgery can certainly be one of the more lucrative branches of medicine. As well as theatre time, consultants will need to run clinics and ward rounds and also spend an increasing amount of time undertaking managerial-type roles. The duties of a surgeon are now formally outlined in a booklet published by the Royal College of Surgeons called *Good Surgical Practice*.

21.3 Training

The training programme in surgery is intensive. This may not suit those with other commitments and interests outside medicine. Flexible training can be arranged through the regional deaneries for those people who meet certain criteria. Other options include part-time training and job sharing. Obviously these programmes would involve more time spent at each level of the career pathway.

The surgical training pathway has recently undergone significant change. Prior to 2005 the pathway from medical school graduation progressed through the pre-registration house officer (PRHO) year and then the senior house officer (SHO) years during which the trainee would have to pass the MRCS examination to become a Member of the Royal College of Surgeons. The SHO years were known as basic surgical training years and would last a minimum of 2 years but sometimes several more. On completion of basic surgical training, a trainee applied for a post at the higher surgical training (HST) level in one of the surgical specialties listed in the box below. During this period the trainee would be a specialist registrar (SpR) and this period of training lasted for 5 or 6 years. After about 4 years of HST the trainee was eligible to take the intercollegiate specialty examination and this led to the award of the Fellowship of the Royal College of Surgeons (FRCS) diploma in the trainee's surgical specialty. At the end of this programme of training the trainee would gain the Certificate of Completion of Specialist Training (CCST) and the qualified surgeon could then enter the General Medical Council's (GMC) Specialist Register and apply for a post as a consultant. There were several stages of competitive entry in this old programme and consequently trainees spent time enhancing their CVs in order to compete for their next promotion. Often trainees spent time in research or clinical posts that provided specialist experience. Many surgical trainees undertook a period of research for 1–3 years to obtain a higher degree (MSc, MD, MS, PhD) either before or during the HST programme. Most of the current consultants trained under this scheme and some of the names for the posts are still used interchangeably with the new names.

In 2005 a new training programme was initiated. All medical training is undergoing a radical transformation; these changes are currently evolving and up-to-date information is available on the Modernizing Medical Careers (MMC) website (www.mmc.nhs.uk). Instead of PRHO posts, medical school graduates now proceed into a Foundation Year 1 (FY1) post (similar to a PRHO post). They will then enter a Foundation Year 2 (FY2) post. These posts will provide broad training and trainees will have to demonstrate clinical competence and other work-related skills that will be assessed in a number of different ways. The first new-style trainees finished their FY2 in August 2007. During the FY2 year trainees will have to make a decision about which area of medicine they want to pursue: medicine, surgery, general practice, etc. If accepted onto a training programme, the trainee will then spend the first 2 or 3 years in a variety of related specialties to their chosen field. During this period the trainee will be assessed on an annual basis. The trainee will then apply via local or national selection for their HST in their chosen specialty for 5 or 6 years before being eligible to sit the specialty exam and complete their training. At this point trainees will be able to apply for a consultant post. The idea behind these changes is to streamline medical training, remove unnecessary hurdles and allow good candidates to proceed rapidly to consultant level. This will shorten post-qualification training from 9–12 years to 7 or 8 years for most surgical specialties. In some of the surgical specialties there is run-through training from finishing the Foundation Programme to consultant. This means that once you are appointed to a training programme after FY2, provided you complete the competency-based annual assessments, you will progress through training in that field without further interviews or selection processes. The next interview will be for a consultant post. Orthopaedics and neurosurgery currently offer this style of training.

Separate training programmes have been set up for those trainees who have an interest in an academic career. Those with an interest in research or teaching can apply for an academic training post (from FY2 onwards) in their specialty of choice (medicine, surgery or general practice). This programme will contain similar clinical training but also dedicated protected time for research and teaching. Academic trainees will be expected to temporarily leave clinical training in order to do 3 years research for a PhD (or equivalent).

For all surgical specialties, training is now recorded online using the Intercollegiate Surgical Curriculum Programme (ISCP) (www.iscp.ac.uk). This is a central website for keeping a logbook of surgical activity, recording assessments and maintaining a portfolio of surgical training. This site is used at the Annual Review of Competence Progression (ARCP) meetings, which determine progression through the training years. Poor performance may result in repeating a year or being offered targeted training.

Surgical specialties

- Breast
- Cardiothoracic: heart and chest
- General: gastrointestinal system
- Neurosurgery: brain and spine
- Oral and maxillofacial: teeth and face
- Orthopaedic: bones and joints
- Otolaryngology: ear, nose and throat
- Paediatrics: children
- Plastic surgery: reconstructive, cosmetic
- Urology: kidney, bladder, prostate
- Vascular: blood vessels

21.4 The surgical exams and courses

The Member of the Royal College of Surgeons (MRCS) examination is currently taken during either the Foundation or core training years (the 2 years after FY2). Surgical trainees will also continue to be required to have successfully completed an approved basic surgical skills (BSS) course. The MRCS is currently split into two parts: Part A consists of two multiple-choice papers; Part B comprises an OSCE (Objective Structured Clinical Exercise) exam (examining actors and clinical information). Two other courses, the ATLS (Advanced Trauma and Life Support) and CCrISP (Care of the Critically Ill Surgical Patient), are also recommended as part of training.

21.5 The job

One of the main preconceptions about surgery is that surgeons spend all their time operating. Generally speaking, this only occupies around a quarter of the working week. A surgeon will have patients on the ward, either waiting for their operation (preop) or having had the procedure carried out (postop). The surgeon will see these patients on a daily ward round. Another activity is seeing patients in the outpatients' clinic, where people who have surgical conditions are seen after being referred by their GP. We have outlined a typical day of a consultant surgeon below.

A day in the life of a consultant surgeon

The day usually starts at 8 a.m. with a ward round. All the patients in a hospital are under the care of a consultant, and surgery is not an exception.

He or she will see the patients under his or her care and also those who have been admitted as emergencies. Management plans need to be decided for all the patients, which can then be carried out following the ward round. Some of the patients might be very unwell or require complex investigations. Other patients will have arrived that morning for routine or planned surgical procedures. Each of these patients will be seen before the operation. Some of the patients will be recovering after their operation, some staying for up to 2 weeks, and some will be well enough to be discharged home.

On this day, after the ward round, the surgeon will go to the operating theatre for the list, which is likely to last around 3 hours. There will be patients having different types of operations, some short cases and some long and difficult procedures. The consultant will be assisted by other trainee surgeons on the team and one of the responsibilities is the training of these junior doctors. After the operating list, during lunchtime, there is usually a meeting to attend. This could be a radiology meeting, where the X-rays of patients are reviewed, or possibly an audit meeting or teaching session.

This typical day involves an outpatient clinic in the afternoon. The clinic involves seeing patients, asking about their symptoms and examining them, and possibly making a diagnosis. The patient might then require surgery and be put on the waiting list, or might be treated with medications. You might have to tell a patient good or bad news depending on the condition and prognosis (outlook).

Every fifth night you will need to be on-call, where patients who are unwell are admitted to hospital, either referred from GPs or from the casualty department. The patients may be very sick, and could require an urgent operation. This can be very hectic if lots of patients turn up at once. You will also have other responsibilities.

- Teaching medical students and the other doctors on the firm.
- Research: investigating new or existing modes and outcomes of surgery.
- Audit: ensuring that the work being carried out in the hospital is being done to an acceptable standard.
- Paperwork: writing notes, reports or letters to GPs and other doctors.

21.6 The options

Several decades ago, a surgeon was able to perform many different operations. It was not unusual for a surgeon to operate on breast, bowel, vascular and urological problems. In the modern era surgeons tend to be less general and focus on a particular area, a specialty. Even the gastrointestinal tract has been split into smaller areas and it is common for a surgeon to become a specialist in either upper or lower gastrointestinal operations.

21.7 Women in surgery

Women now comprise 6% of consultant surgeons and 22% of surgical trainees, and these numbers are growing. A group called Women in Surgery (WinS) was set up by the Royal College of Surgeons in September 1991 (www.surgicalcareers.rcseng.ac.uk/wins); it was formerly known as Women in Surgical Training. The aim of WinS is to promote surgery as a career for women and to enable women who have chosen a career in surgery to realize their professional goals.

21.8 Training abroad

Under the MRCS regulations only those posts approved by the surgical royal colleges of England, Edinburgh, Glasgow and Ireland are recognized as entry requirements for the examination along with other posts stated in the regulations.

21.9 Flexible training

This is possible in surgery and is becoming more common, although less so than in other specialties within medicine. The training period must be approved by the specific royal college before commencement. You can get advice on flexible training from the college's flexible training adviser, who can be contacted via the training board by letter, by email at careers@rcseng. ac.uk, or by telephone on 020 74053474.

21.10 Further information

An excellent source of information is the surgical careers day held several times a year at the Royal College of Surgeons in London. There are guest speakers from every step of the surgical career pathway. Each speaker is then subjected to a question and answer session. The day concludes with a tour of the college and a surgical skills session. Each student also receives an information pack about CV skills and the career pathway.

21.11 The surgical specialties

Cardiothoracic

As the name suggests this field deals with the heart and chest and includes the famous coronary artery bypass graft (to bypass blocked arteries that supply the heart), replacing heart valves, heart transplants, repairing inherited heart defects in children, and some operations for victims of chest trauma. The cardiothoracic surgeon also operates on the lungs. This is very demanding work. Most of the operations by their nature are carried out on people who are not very fit and this brings associated risks. Cardiothoracic surgeons work closely with cardiologists (medical heart specialists) and respiratory physicians (lung specialists) who will refer patients for surgery and perform preoperative assessments and investigations. This is a challenging field of surgery that requires significant commitment.

ENT surgery/otolaryngology

ENT is the popular way of saying 'otorhinolaryngology', or head and neck surgery. Although you are working on just one small part of the body, there is a huge amount of skill required. The job involves repairing disorders of hearing, smell, taste, and speech and language. Although you will be performing a wide range of operations, there are also a lot of patients to be seen in the outpatient clinic. One of the joys of ENT is a chance to play with some of the weird and wonderful technology, such as microscopes and endoscope cameras to look into the body. A good ENT surgeon will be able to listen to patients' problems, have good management skills, good manual and technical skills, and be able to work as part of a multidisciplinary team.

General surgery

A decade ago, a general surgeon would operate on the major blood vessels, the breast and the bowels – quite a job. Now the specialty is subspecializing, but all surgeons still initially train in all those areas. Consultant general surgeons are usually practitioners in one of these subspecialty areas and also take responsibility for acute general surgical take. The practical elements and enjoyment of the practical tasks are probably the main attractions to any surgical specialty. The challenge is to perform the repeated practical task to an even higher degree of excellence. Nonetheless, skilful decision-making about patient management and meticulous postoperative care also provide challenges and their own rewards. A good general surgeon will be able to undertake responsibilities, have good manual dexterity, good organizational ability, and be physically fit!

Although the training to become a general surgeon is the same at the registrar level, most consultant surgeons then specialize in one area of:
- gastrointestinal (bowel) surgery
- breast surgery
- vascular surgery.

Gastrointestinal surgeons operate on conditions such as cancer of the colon or stomach ulceration. Many patients are admitted to hospital on-call with problems such as a perforated bowel. These patients can become extremely unwell in a short period of time and although medical management can help, an operation is usually necessary.

Breast surgeons deal with both benign and cancerous diseases of the breast, seeing patients in clinic and, following a biopsy, perform a relevant operation.

Vascular surgeons deal with blood vessel disease, such as blockages and burst vessels. Again, many patients attend the hospital extremely unwell and require intensive treatment both before and after surgery.

Maxillofacial surgery

This is almost a separate field. Most hospital maxillofacial surgeons have dual qualifications in dentistry and medicine. Most have done a dentistry degree first and then want to pursue a career in more complex surgery around the mouth and face. This surgery now overlaps with ENT and plastic surgery to some degree. These surgeons also see trauma to the facial bones and perform more complicated dental procedures. Most dentists get some experience in a maxillofacial unit as part of their training.

Neurosurgery

Neurosurgeons operate on the nervous system, which encompasses both the brain and the spinal cord. They diagnose and treat a variety of diseases that can affect it. Neurological problems are common and make up to one-quarter of all emergency hospital admissions. Neurosurgeons do not just operate; they also look after the intensive-care management and rehabilitation of patients with disorders affecting the brain and skull, spine, and nervous system. The subspecialties include spinal surgery, treatment for epilepsy and the care of children. Following recent advances in technology, for example in computed tomography (CT) and magnetic resonance imaging (MRI), many more neurological conditions are curable, for example head trauma and spinal injuries. The qualities required include a caring attitude, ability to work in a team, honesty, reliability, understanding of one's limitations, good communication skills and organizational ability.

Orthopaedic and trauma surgery

Elective orthopaedic surgery takes place in most district general hospitals, making it one of the largest of the specialties within surgery. The specialty has certainly seen significant changes in the last two decades, with the advent of new instruments and techniques, for example minimally invasive surgery. There is now a spectrum of subspecialties available, ranging from joint replacements in hips and knees to microvascular surgery. The specialty is well balanced, with routine operating cases complemented by a large number of trauma cases, which can be very exciting and rewarding. Working closely with other therapists (e.g. physiotherapy) and other specialties makes this a dynamic subject. The last few years have also seen major developments in the management of trauma patients, with an increasing number of injuries being treated operatively, enabling more rapid patient rehabilitation. The qualities required are good manual dexterity, ability to learn biomechanical and biological concepts, dedication and enthusiasm, good spatial awareness to cope with procedures under X-ray control, and teamwork.

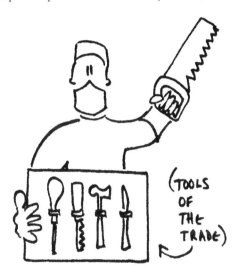

Career paths: orthopaedics

Paediatric surgery

This specialty involves a diverse workload that encroaches onto many other specialties, for example eyes and plastic and orthopaedic surgery. The main areas of surgery are trauma, intestinal and neonatal surgery. As a paediatric surgeon, you will work closely with GPs and other hospital doctors. There is limited opportunity for private practice. On-call commitments can vary but the emergency workload is interesting and never routine. It is a rewarding but busy career choice. Patience and good surgical techniques are required for this specialty, as are good communication and decision-making skills as you must support the parents as well as the child.

Plastic surgery

A broad-ranging specialty that also assists many other specialties, for example cleft lip and palate surgery, breast reconstructive surgery, craniofacial surgery, limb reconstruction from either trauma or congenital abnormality, urogenital surgery in conjunction with the urologist (see below), and treating conditions of the skin. There is also cosmetic surgery, for example of the breast and face. Hand surgery can also form some of the workload, with a significant amount of congenital and traumatic problems. Plastic surgery is a truly dynamic specialty and encourages basic scientific and clinical research. The work is challenging, exciting and rewarding. A good plastic surgeon would have a high level of manual dexterity and technical skill, an enquiring mind and lateral thinking ability, and an understanding of the principles of audit and evidence-based medicine.

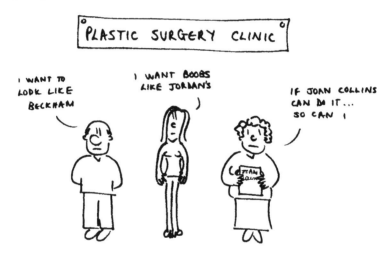

Urology

This is a very dynamic specialty involving surgery of the kidney, bladder and genitourinary system. Many changes have occurred recently with the introduction of minimally invasive techniques. There is a good variety of emergency work and routine operations. Subspecialties include andrology (male hormone treatments), endo-urology (endoscopic treatments, i.e. using probes and scopes), female urology, neuro-urology, oncological urology (cancer), paediatric urology and reconstructive urology. You will see patients with a wide breadth of pathology, including urinary tract stone disease, infections, and malignancy. Three of the most predominant male cancers are urological: prostate, bladder and kidney cancers. In the younger male age group, testicular cancer is number one of this group of cancers. There is an interesting range of surgical skills required, both endoscopic and open, and urology has lots of new technology in its repertoire. If people are particularly interested, they can also extend their practice outside conventional boundaries, for example performing transrectal (via the patient's bottom) ultrasound scans and biopsies. Because most departments are relatively small in respect of consultant numbers, there may be fairly frequent on-call sessions, but urology on-call is not arduous and there is an increasing trend to cross-cover with neighbouring hospitals to reduce the on-call frequency. The qualities required are good patient and colleague communication, ability to work in a team, and good manual dexterity demonstrated by both open and endoscopic operative skills.

21.12 Summary

Surgery is a diverse, rewarding but demanding career. It offers the opportunity to combine manual practical skills with medical treatments. The results of surgery in patients provides rapid feedback which is a constant challenge to improve. New technology is constantly being implemented and procedures become more and more complex and innovative. Training in surgery has been significantly condensed in recent years and working patterns and attitudes improved.

PERSONAL VIEW   *Sir Peter Morris*

Although I only decided to do medicine 6 months or so before I was due to go to university, I was quite sure, having made the decision to enter medicine rather than engineering, that I wanted to be a surgeon. To some extent this decision was influenced by reading a biography of Henry Cushing, the famous neurosurgeon in Boston in the 1930s, and also to some extent by the fact that, as a good ball player, I liked doing things with my hands.

The 6 years at medical school at the University of Melbourne were the best years of my life. I was a reasonable student but had lots of interests outside medicine. Nevertheless, my ambition to be a surgeon never changed. After graduation and completing my house jobs, I spent a further 3 years as a surgical resident at St Vincent's Hospital, Melbourne. It was during those several years that I had a lucky break. Dr Claude Welsh, a famous surgeon

(continued)

(*Continued*)

from the Massachusetts General Hospital (MGH) in Boston, came to St Vincent's as a visiting professor. In those days a visiting professor came for several months and operated most days on complex cases saved up for the great man by the surgical staff of the hospital. I was fortunate enough to be selected as his surgical registrar during his time in Melbourne, which meant that I was with him all day, every day, seeing patients, doing ward rounds and operating with him. He was an inspiration as a surgeon: he never raised his voice, said please and thank you to everyone, even in the operating room, and yet achieved outstanding results in the complex surgical cases he had been asked to tackle. He was my ideal surgeon and the experience reinforced not only my resolve to be a surgeon but also my concept of the ideal behaviour of a practising surgeon. After he left we kept in touch and several years later I was to go to the USA and the MGH at his request. My surgical training started in Australia, after which I went to the UK for just over 2 years before going to Boston, first as a senior resident in surgery and then as a junior staff man and research fellow at Harvard Medical School. As an aside, I did spend 6 months in general practice before leaving for the UK, in order to save some money for the trip, and I thoroughly enjoyed this experience.

I had an excellent training in the UK, in London and especially in Southampton where I received an enormous amount of supervised operative experience under the tutelage of Mr Tom Rowntree. Moving to the USA was another major influence on my career, for not only did I learn within the huge department of surgery at the MGH that there were many ways of tackling a given operation, but also I was exposed to research for the first time. Initially I worked on the immunology of inflammation and infection but later switched to the immunology of transplantation, with a particular interest in tissue matching, a science in its infancy at that time. This experience made me sure that I wished to pursue a career in academic surgery, not only performing surgery but also doing research in areas of relevance to my clinical practice. Another lucky break followed when, just before I was due to return to Australia, I was asked by David Hume, the famous pioneer transplant surgeon, to join his department at Richmond, Virginia. Here he had established the largest transplant unit in the world at that time, and he wanted me to set up a tissue typing laboratory for the unit. This I did over a 7-month period as that was all the time I could give him before returning to Australia. This was another extraordinary experience in that I achieved what I had been asked to do but was also able to make some major contributions to the field of tissue matching using samples that Hume had preserved from the time of his first transplant.

On return to the University of Melbourne, I was a lecturer in the Department of Surgery with wide-ranging clinical responsibilities in general surgery and transplantation. One must realize that in those days we were trained as true general surgeons. I also started the transplantation research laboratories and set up another tissue typing laboratory, the first in Australia. After a very successful and enjoyable 7 years in Melbourne, by which time I had gone from lecturer to senior lecturer and finally reader in surgery, I was invited to Oxford University as the Nuffield Professor of Surgery and Chairmanship of the department at the ripe old age of 39. It was a great move in many ways as I was able to set up a transplant and vascular unit, the two specialties I eventually concentrated on. Research took off rapidly as six of my technicians came to Oxford with me, and so the laboratories were up and running quickly and the department never looked back.

So why be a surgeon? Certainly, if I had my time all over again, I have not the slightest doubt that I would do surgery once more. In surgical practice, in contrast to many other disciplines, you have the opportunity of curing a patient's problems by a properly selected and carefully done operation. There is nothing quite so rewarding!

Surgery has changed enormously over my career – many operations have disappeared completely as new medical treatments have appeared (e.g. peptic ulcer surgery), while many new operations have appeared, for example laparoscopic cholecystectomy (removal of the gallbladder by keyhole surgery). I have no doubt that change will continue to occur, especially in the age of molecular biology, which will have an impact on surgical practice just as in medicine generally. But surgery will remain a marvellous discipline in which to specialize, particularly if you remember that a surgeon is a physician who operates.

Chapter 22 **Working abroad**

Although different models of healthcare exist around the world, all of them require doctors. This means it is possible for doctors to travel and work in other parts of the world. The British medical degree is well respected around the world, and language is often the only limiting factor as to choice of location. A couple of decades ago, taking time out from your training as a junior doctor was frowned upon and could have harmed career progression. This culture has changed and most employers now agree that working abroad can broaden a doctor's experience and it tends to be considered more favourably. This has seen increasing numbers of doctors spending time during their junior years in foreign places. There are many reasons for choosing to spend some of your training abroad or even to move permanently; other countries may offer different experiences, fairer climates or a better work/life balance. Although some doctors choose to move to Western countries with similar healthcare structures, many doctors choose to work in poorer countries and often volunteer. In general, since the introduction of Modernizing Medical Careers (MMC), there appears to be concern as to whether it will be as easy to venture abroad due to the shortened and more structured training.

After deciding to work abroad, you must then decide where, when and what to do. This involves researching the countries, hospitals and jobs, and talking to your senior colleagues as well as emailing and faxing potential hospitals. We list the advantages and disadvantages of working abroad in the box below.

Advantages to working abroad
- Change of scene
- Cultural experience
- Opportunity to travel

The Essential Guide to Becoming a Doctor, 3rd edition. © Adrian Blundell, Richard Harrison and Benjamin Turney. Published 2011 by Blackwell Publishing Ltd.

- Meet new people
- Learn new skills
- Break from the career ladder
- Experience different healthcare system
- Experience different pathology
- Volunteer

Disadvantages to working abroad
- Potential disruption to career path
- Leaving family and loved ones
- Problems applying and being interviewed for positions back home
- Organizing the paperwork
- Potential expense

22.1 Planning

Organizing the trip usually takes several months and it is worth being well prepared. It is essential to first realize your own objectives for wanting to work abroad and spend time researching the possible options. Try to speak to doctors who have 'been there and done that'. Once a location has been decided, there are two choices: organize the job yourself or use an agency. Agencies can take a lot of the hassle out of finding a placement. Some of them have national interviews at certain times of the year in order to recruit. They offer incentives, such as free flights and insurance, but often the jobs are in more isolated locations, where recruitment has proved difficult from local graduates.

As an alternative to using an agency, contact the human resources department of hospitals directly; most of the hospitals will have internet sites. Send a copy of your CV with a covering letter to the medical staffing department and see what happens. It is always worthwhile making a follow-up phone call to ensure they have received your CV and also to discuss opportunities in person. Medical staffing should then tell you the process of when the jobs become available and how to apply. Then you must finalize details of the actual job and salary; make sure you clarify that the job is of a suitable seniority, that your experience is adequate and confirm a salary. Many jobs are advertised on the web, either by the individual hospital or even by the regional health authority; in some instances it is possible to do a job search for the whole region for the particular specialty that appeals, and then apply online. It is also worth browsing the careers section in the *British Medical Journal* each week.

Your future employer will require various documentation. Firstly, check if the country you will be working in requires a visa. Again this can take some sorting, so it is worth considering early on. Most embassies issue visas by post but it can take 1–2 months. You also need to make sure your passport is valid for the full time you are abroad. Most developed countries will require evidence of your health status. This will, at the minimum, mean proof of your hepatitis status and other vaccines but you may also need a chest radiograph and HIV status. Don't forget that for some countries you may need further immunizations.

Travel insurance is necessary and each individual request will be different, depending on length of stay, which country, possible procedures performed, accommodation type, etc. A Certificate of Good Standing (which states that no complaints have been made regarding your practice), available from the General Medical Council (GMC), is requested by most employers. Copies of your actual GMC certificate, CV, references and university degree may also be required (and original documentation can be asked for). Another factor to be considered is your NHS pension. Depending on your length of service, this may merely be frozen during your trip, but in some circumstances it may be cancelled. Contact the pension agency (through your employer) and explore the options.

On arrival at your destination, you must register with the local medical board. Temporary registration is usually not a problem and your employer should have made them aware of your imminent arrival. Remember, all of the above will incur costs, so bear this in mind when budgeting and deciding on flight arrangements. Before leaving check with your indemnity insurance company that you will be covered abroad and make alternative arrangements if not.

The final consideration is to think about the possible implications for your future career. Ideally, only accept positions that will be recognized towards your training. For further information browse the checklist on the support4doctors website (www.support4doctors.org/advice.asp?id=199).

22.2 When to go: the past

Traditionally, the majority of medical graduates travelled abroad at some point during their first 2 years as a senior house officer. It was important to complete the pre-registration house officer (PRHO) year as most countries expected full registration with the GMC. Most packed their bags immediately after finishing as a PRHO, and spent between 6 months and 2 years abroad (some stayed and never returned!). It was also possible to work abroad at other natural career breaks, such as between SHO and SpR and SpR and consultant. It was also possible to spend part of your registrar training abroad and some doctors even took up locum consultant posts before settling into their specialty back home. There is a minority of practitioners who remain abroad, some meeting lifelong partners and others finding the lure of the beach too great. The focus of this chapter is for those thinking of spending a short time in a different country. In summary, it was actually possible to work abroad during any part of your medical life but this did depend on your career choice and your examination timetable.

22.3 When to go: the future

With the introduction of MMC, the attitudes and timing for working abroad have changed somewhat. Because of the introduction of the 2-year Foundation Programme, very few doctors now move abroad after their first year. Although not impossible to change countries for the FY2 year (see Personal view by Emma Lane), this is very rare and for good reason: the idea of the foundation training is based on a 2-year programme. Doctors considering moving after their FY1 year would need to be certain that the job abroad enabled completion of the appropriate competencies otherwise they would struggle to return to the UK system. A natural break now is following the Foundation Programme and prior to specialty training. Unfortunately, due to the system being in its infancy, anecdotally there has been concern about future career prospects and so many trainees have decided against moving abroad. On the other hand, after the MTAS fiasco (see Chapter 15), some excellent trainees found themselves unable to obtain employment and so moved abroad with the idea of completing their training abroad. Although appearing more difficult than during previous training structures, if you are keen to work abroad then the experience should be valuable, so do go.

22.4 Where to go

There are two options: study medicine in the Western world, with similar technology and healthcare systems as the UK, or travel to a developing country. Colleagues choosing the latter have generally found themselves working more alone and at times with greater responsibility (see Personal view by Julian Boullin). The other big decision is whether to spend time in an English-speaking country or not. This will really depend on your language ability.

Europe

While it is possible to work in Europe, this will be extremely difficult without a firm grasp of the local language. The advantage of Europe is the proximity and recognition of the British medical qualification. This means it is possible to work with confirmation of your competency provided by the GMC and without the need for a work permit. Basically doctors can move freely within the European Union as long as they are a citizen of a member state and have completed medical training in a member state. Language can be a problem; an A level in the subject is likely to be the minimal requirement necessary. Some doctors do attend language classes to assist them while abroad. While there are no formal language examinations, it is important to notify your future employers of your level of ability. Some hospitals do run exchange schemes and these are often advertised in the *BMJ* careers section. The advantage of being from the UK is that, in most of the European countries where you might work, English is spoken fluently, and many of the medical journals are also published in English.

Further information regarding working in each of the EU countries can be found in the booklet *Opportunities for doctors in the European Economic Area*, which can be found on the BMA website.

Australasia

The majority of UK graduates head off to seek warmer climates down under. With no language barrier, similar healthcare systems and plenty of adventure activities, it is easy to understand why. Certainly at ST1/ST2, there are lots of opportunities, especially in emergency medicine and relief work (covering doctors on annual leave). At ST3 level and above, it can be a little harder and it is often necessary to pass further local exams.

There are some differences that need to be noted. Firstly, the grading of a doctor is slightly different. The hierarchy runs: consultant, advanced trainee registrar, basic trainee registrar, resident medical officer (RMO) (or hospital medical officer, HMO) and intern. The new training structure in the UK is more in line with the Australian system than the previous career ladder, so that FY1 corresponds to intern, FY2 to RMO, ST1/ST2 to basic trainee registrar, and ST3+ to advanced trainee registrar.

The other main differences are the working patterns and wages. Each hospital will have individualized rotas but in general the hours are less than in the UK, and instead of receiving a standard wage it is common practice to complete time-sheets. In this way a doctor gets paid for the actual hours worked, and so if you are working nights or working a bank holiday, your pay reflects this. Do be aware that many of the jobs offered are in rural places where it is difficult to recruit local graduates.

USA

A much smaller number of graduates from the UK end up working in the USA compared with Europe and Australasia. Although there is no obvious language barrier, the healthcare systems differ considerably and further examinations are required for the privilege. Most UK doctors who go to the USA have family connections and it is wise to make the decision to go early during your university years. International medical graduates (IMGs) need certification from the Educational Commission for Foreign Medical Graduates (ECFMG) in order to be eligible to enrol in a residency programme and then be able to apply for licensure to practice medicine. This process can be both time-consuming and expensive. It also involves completing a further qualification called the United States Medical Licensing Examination (USMLE). This consists of three steps and some of the process can only be carried out on US soil, leading to further expense.

Job allocation is done by a matching scheme, similar to that used by some of the universities in the UK. The jobs commence in July, which is not in line with British positions, and so could lead to some forced travel time or locum work. The other difficulty may be obtaining a visa and so advanced preparation is more essential than for moving to Australasia. As already mentioned, the healthcare systems are different, and so are working practices. The European Working Time Directive (as its name suggests) does not apply to the USA. The work may well be more intensive and working long hours is common. With private healthcare many patients have more extensive investigations to achieve a diagnosis. Less emphasis on bedside clinical skills and more reliance on technology can be disappointing for some clinicians, as can the increased litigation that can ensue.

As the working practices differ across the Atlantic, it would be sensible to organize an elective placement or observership in order to test the water. This will give you the opportunity to experience the American way before being committed to any contract or working future. Further information can be found in the BMA booklet *Guide to Working Abroad* (see the BMA website).

It is frequently possible for doctors to travel and work in other parts of the world

The developing world

Working in the developing world tends to involve working on a voluntary basis, although this does not mean the work is any easier to obtain; there is often great competition for places and it is not unusual to be placed on a waiting list. One of the better-known agencies is Medicins Sans Frontières. If you are accepted, work will normally be offered for approximately 12 months, and many of these groups send doctors to a great variety of destinations. Although there is often no formal wage, set-up costs and living expenses are usually covered. Other funding be available for doctors wishing to spend time doing voluntary work. It is a case of trying as many different sources as possible. Write to local companies, charities, family, friends, or even partake in a sponsored event. Although it may be possible to arrange work in the developing world independently, the majority of doctors will use an agency. In view of the type of work, the positions are often for more experienced doctors. Further information can be found in the BMA booklet *Guide to Working Abroad* (see the BMA website).

Working abroad checklist

- Valid passport
- Relevant visa
- Immunization records
- Occupational health report
- Certificate of Good Standing
- Travel insurance
- Indemnity cover
- Stethoscope
- *British National Formulary*
- Medical supplies
- Copies of all relevant documents (scan and email documents to yourself and family)
- Medical books

22.5 Other options

All work and no play may make for a dull life. Working abroad is a great opportunity to experience a different culture and many doctors spend some of their spare time travelling. Although previously frowned upon by potential employers, most now realize that time spent away can be useful and character building. It is not essential to work in a hospital or general practice while away. A minority fancy a more adventurous time and embark on journeys aboard cruise ships or even round-the-world yacht races. Most of us have heard of the flying doctors in Australia, but there are many less developed countries that also rely on these services. Information about these activities can be found on the internet or in medical journals. To take part in sailing trips or mountain treks as the medical adviser will entail funding. This again has to be taken into consideration when taking account of your financial situation. Other companies may arrange working abroad seminars, so keep an eye out in the national journals.

22.6 Summary

Although potentially more difficult following the introduction of the Foundation Programme and run-through training, there will still be possibilities for working abroad for those who wish. The best advice is to try to plan well ahead. It is often possible to organize your trip single-handedly; most doctors travel with friends or partners but, if you are alone, do not be put off. Most of the hospitals in Australasia have large communities of British medical staff, many of whom have emigrated. The internet is a vast source of knowledge for those arranging foreign travel and work. We have included some useful internet addresses at the end of the book. Medical newspapers and journals also have jobs advertised. The other important point to remember is that no matter where you have chosen to visit, other doctors will have been there before. Ask for their hints and tips and it may help you decide and also save some time.

PERSONAL VIEW   *Emma Lane*

Frustrated by the constraints of the UK training scheme and struggling with my itchy feet, I decided to ignore the advice of my seniors who recommended to go abroad after I had completed the Foundation Programme and instead listened to my headstrong self, broke free and applied to do my FY2 year in New Zealand. It is certainly not common for a doctor to leave their UK post after FY1 and I was warned of its potentially detrimental effect on my further training. In reality I have found that doctors on both sides of the world are fully supporting my career decision and so far everything appears to be running smoothly.

Even the actual paperwork seemed a little too easy to be true. I found a document entitled *Application for FY2 overseas* complete with a checklist of requirements and a deadline for applications. Each deanery has its own rules and regulations and should have an equivalent document. My first step was

(continued)

(*Continued*)

to find a job. I rang an agency that was advertised in the *BMJ*, sent them my CV and within a week was being asked what rotations I would like to do and when I wanted to start! I had to ensure I had a good balance of jobs, get the hospital in New Zealand to sign some papers to say they would support my educational needs, and send the documents with a covering letter to the head of the deanery. The agency sorted out all the correspondence and most of the paperwork including work permits and visas. I sent everything off and the next thing I knew I was writing a letter resigning from my FY2 post in England. In terms of completing assessments, the deanery has rearranged my deadline schedule to fit in with my rotations here in New Zealand. The hospitals in New Zealand are keen for more UK graduates to work here so are doing everything they can to make it possible to do an FY2 accredited year here.

So, now I'm here, what's it like? The hospitals themselves are fairly similar to those in the UK, as are standards of practice. There are, however, a number of differences and it's interesting to see how a different health system functions. For example, some medications in New Zealand are government subsidized and some are not, meaning you can't always discharge your patients on the medication you want to as it is too expensive for the patient. It definitely allows you to appreciate the NHS!

The lifestyle here is amazing. The people in New Zealand work to live, as opposed to the live to work attitude that seems to be developing in the UK. My weekends are spent exploring the country and I have found that New Zealand definitely lives up to its reputation as an adventure playground. Adrenaline-fuelled activities are never far away: sky-diving, bungee jumping, caving, surfing, rafting; you name it, I've done it! Aside from adventure, the cost of living here is much cheaper so I have found myself with a greater disposable income than previously. At least, that was until I discovered New World wines: New Zealand is relatively young in the world of wine but vineyards are abundant and tastings are usually free (bottles, however, unfortunately not!). The only real downside to the country is that it is ever so far away from the rest of the world. If I was only here for a year or two it's perfect, and if it were closer to home I wouldn't think twice about staying.

Spending a year here gives you a whole new perspective on life and work, and I would highly recommend the experience. In terms of when to go, most people go between FY2 and ST1, which is a natural break and works well. I've found that making the year count as FY2 gives you an effective year out without actually taking time out of a training scheme. This means that if you wanted you could feasibly take another year out to have fun and get different experiences without taking more than a year out of a training scheme. Why would you pass up on that?!

PERSONAL VIEW *Julian Boullin*

Following on from house jobs, like many of my friends, I decided that I would like to spend some time working abroad. Unlike most of them, I did not go to Australasia. Although very tempting, I wanted to use this opportunity to do something a little different and in my mind more challenging. I had travelled to East Africa during my student holidays and felt that I wanted to return to this part of the world as a qualified doctor. I went to a meeting entitled 'Doctors Working Abroad' at the Royal Geographic Society and picked up a leaflet detailing working as a volunteer for the African Medical Research Foundation (AMREF) in their flying doctors service. I wrote to the head of emergency services at AMREF enclosing my curriculum vitae and outlining why I wanted the posting, and was very lucky to be offered a job as a flight physician.

After completing 6 months of accident and emergency in this country, I spent three fantastic months based in Nairobi, Kenya. Like many jobs in Africa I had to find funding myself. The major expense was the flight but once this was paid for, living expenses were not too great. I travelled to Kenya as a (pre-MMC) senior house officer, which meant that I was relatively junior. The job would ideally suit a trainee after completion of the Acute Care Common Stem or during speciality training.

My days were spent going on air evacuations during daylight hours. On receiving a call-out, a pilot, nurse and I loaded up a small aircraft with all the necessary equipment including that to resuscitate and ventilate a patient if required. We then took off from the airport at which we were based. Roughly two-thirds of the patients were covered by private insurance and this helped fund the 'free' evacuations. There was a vast range of call-outs, from road traffic accidents to acute medical emergencies, including tropical diseases. Some days we would fly and pick up a tourist with a simple leg injury or fever; other times we would transfer critically unwell patients usually from a small local hospital, back to Nairobi where the only intensive-care facilities are available. On one occasion we landed on a dusty airstrip on the border of Sudan to find a young Dutch missionary woman only just breathing, lying in the back of a jeep, suffering from complicated malaria.

As well as seeing a wide variety of interesting cases, the other side to the job was the opportunity to see the beautiful land of East Africa, often from the air. Flights lasted anything from half an hour to 4 hours. I remember flying over snow-topped Kilimanjaro, then having to sweep over our landing strip in a game park several times in order to clear the zebra and wildebeest before

(continued)

(*Continued*)

we could land. During my visit I was very fortunate to accompany a group of business executives who requested a stand-by doctor, pilot and plane during their safari. This meant a free luxury trip with game drives, complete with hot-air balloon trip at sunrise and champagne breakfast!

On the downside it could be lonely. This was helped by meeting people who lived in Nairobi, both locals and of course the ever friendly ex-pats who had made their homes there. Due to the current crime levels in the city, walking anywhere after dark was not advised. This meant getting around using taxis or taking lifts with new-found friends. The crime level never caused me any problems but it is essential to take care and be extra vigilant, especially if travelling alone.

Some days there were no evacuations, although you still needed to be available. This was a good time for study, research or to catch up with some old news from back home. The rest of the team were all very welcoming, and it was nice to get to know some very friendly and interesting Kenyans.

Overall this was a unique experience that I shall never forget. All my friends who worked in Australia and New Zealand also had a great time so I could not say this experience was necessarily better. The difference is that newly qualified doctors are not as aware of the possible opportunities in developing countries. The points to note are that the pathology seen can be very different to that in the Western world and the opportunity to develop new skills is probably greater. Remember that it can be lonely and this is not helped by the language barrier, although most people speak at least some English. Also as a more junior doctor, with little experience, it is possible that at times there may be little senior support.

Working in Africa will not be for everyone, but if you wish to work abroad, do bear it in mind.

Appendix

The following is a list of suggested websites where further information can be found. Where possible they are organised under the relevant chapter headings, although there will be overlap. We cannot guarantee the accuracy of the information on each site and do not endorse any of the products or services that may be offered. To gain the most from this list we suggest that you browse and select those areas that you find personally interesting – happy searching!

A challenging career

http://www.dfes.gov.uk/studentsupport/
http://www.gmc-uk.org/
https://medicas.org.uk/
http://www.medlink-uk.com/
http://www.nhscareers.nhs.uk/nhs-knowledge_base/data/5343.html
http://www.premed.org.uk
http://targetjobs.co.uk/career-sectors/medicine

The application procedure

http://www.bbc.co.uk/dna/h2g2/A717527
http://www.medschoolsonline.co.uk/
http://www.newmediamedicine.com/forum/content/
http://www.thestudentroom.co.uk/wiki/A_Rookies_Guide_To_Getting_Into_Medical_School
http://www.ucas.com
http://www.wanttobeadoctor.co.uk/main.php

The Essential Guide to Becoming a Doctor, 3rd edition. © Adrian Blundell, Richard Harrison and Benjamin Turney. Published 2011 by Blackwell Publishing Ltd.

The year out
http://www.bunac.org/
http://www.gapwork.com/
http://www.gapyear.com/
http://www.gapyearjobs.co.uk/
http://www.lattitude.org.uk/
http://www.missionafrica.org.uk/
http://www.payaway.co.uk/
http://www.projecttrust.org.uk/
http://www.teaching-abroad.co.uk/
http://www.travellersworldwide.com/
http://www.work4travel.co.uk/
http://www.yearoutgroup.org/

The interview process
http://www.admissionsforum.net/forumdisplay.php?f=31
http://chemistry.about.com/library/weekly/aa013102a.htm
http://news.bbc.co.uk/1/hi/health/
http://gradschool.about.com/cs/medicalinterview/a/medquest.htm
http://www.health-news.co.uk/
http://www.medical-interviews.co.uk/interview-questions-medical-school-interviews.aspx
http://www.newscientist.com/
http://www.studentdoctor.net/index.asp
http://www.thestudentroom.co.uk/wiki/What_you_should_expect_at_a_medical_school_interview

Over 21s
http://www.medschoolsonline.co.uk/index.php?pageid=141
http://www.nhscareers.nhs.uk/nhs-knowledge_base/data/5343.html

Life at medical school
http://omni.ac.uk/browse/mesh/detail/C0038495L0038495.html
http://www.nus.org.uk/
http://www.studentbmj.com
http://www.studentdoctor.net/index.asp
http://www.studentfreestuff.com/
http://www.studentuk.com
http://www.ukstudentguide.co.uk

The preclinical years

http://omni.ac.uk/browse/mesh/detail/C0038495L0038495.html
http://www.drsref.com.au
http://www.fleshandbones.com/default.cfm
http://www.medal.org/
http://www.med.harvard.edu/AANLIB/home.html
http://www.medicalstudent.com/
http://www.studentdoc.com/
http://www.studentmedics.co.uk/
http://www.visembryo.com/

The clinical years

http://www.ecglibrary.com/ecghome.html
http://www.flash-med.com/Fact_Time.asp
http://www.medical-journals.com/
http://www.merck.com/
http://www.nottingham.ac.uk/pathology/medweb.html
http://www.radiology.co.uk/srs-x/index.htm
http://www.the-mdu.com/studentm/

The elective

http://www.electives.net/
http://www.healthserve.org/elecprep/contents.htm
http://www.medicalstudentelectives.org/
http://www.medicstravel.com/
http://www.rdinfo.org.uk
http://www.rsm.ac.uk/academ/awards/index.php
http://www.worktheworld.co.uk/

Finances

http://www.bma.org.uk/careers/medical_education/student_finance/
http://www.money4medstudents.org/index.asp?id=1
http://www.moneynet.co.uk/student_index.shtml
http://practitioners.studentfinanceengland.co.uk
http://www.slc.co.uk
http://www.studentfinancedirect.co.uk
http://www.studentmoney.org.uk/
http://www.direct.gov.uk/EducationAndLearning/UniversityAndHigherEducation/fs/en

Life as a junior doctor

http://money.guardian.co.uk/work/wageslaves/story/0,11996,714966,00.html

http://www.bma.org.uk

http://www.doh.gov.uk/

http://www.doctors.net.uk/

http://www.medicalprotection.org/medical/united_kingdom/default.aspx

http://www.real-doctors.com/

http://www.thedoctorscoach.co.uk

Career paths

Association for Palliative Medicine: http://www.palliative-medicine.org

Association of Anaesthetists: http://www.aagbi.org

Association of British Neurologists: http://www.theabn.org/

Association of Surgeons of GB and Ireland: http://www.asgbi.org.uk

British Association for A&E Medicine: http://www.baem.org.uk

British Association of Dermatologists: http://www.bad.org.uk

British Association of Occupational Therapists: http://www.cot.co.uk

British Cardiac Society: http://www.bcs.com

British Dietetic Association: http://www.bda.uk.com

British Medical Association: http://www.bma.org.uk

British Nuclear Medicine Society: http://www.bnms.org.uk

British Oncological Association: http://www.boaonline.org.uk

British Orthopaedic Association: http://www.boa.ac.uk

British Pharmacological Society: http://www.bps.ac.uk

British Renal Society: http://www.britishrenal.org/

British Society for Audiology: http://www.thebsa.org.uk/

British Society for Endocrinology: http://www.endocrinology.org/

British Society for Geriatrics: http://www.bgs.org.uk/

British Society for Haematology: http://www.blacksci.co.uk/uk/society/bsh

British Society for Immunology: http://immunology.org/

British Society for Neurophysiology: http://www.bscn.org.uk/links.html

British Society for Rheumatology: http://www.rheumatology.org.uk/

British Society of Gastroenterology: http://www.bsg.org.uk

British Society of Rehabilitation Medicine: http://www.bsrm.co.uk/

British Thoracic Society: http://www.brit-thoracic.org.uk

Diabetes UK: http://www.diabetes.org

Modernising Medical Careers: www.mmc.nhs.uk

RCP Faculty of Pharmaceutical Medicine: http://www.f-pharm-med.org.uk

Royal College of Anaesthetists: http://www.rcoa.ac.uk

Royal College of General Practitioners: http://www.rcgp.org.uk

Royal College of Obstetricians and Gynaecologists: http://www.rcog.org.uk
Royal College of Ophthalmologists: http://www.rcophth.ac.uk
Royal College of Paediatrics and Child Health: http://www.rcpch.ac.uk
Royal College of Pathologists: http://www.rcpath.org/contents.html
Royal College of Physicians: http://www.rcplondon.ac.uk
Royal College of Physicians of Edinburgh: http://www.rcpe.ac.uk
Royal College of Physicians & Surgeons of Glasgow: http://www. rcpsglasg. ac.uk/index.html
Royal College of Psychiatry: http://www.rcpsych.ac.uk
Royal College of Radiologists: http://www.rcrad.org.uk/
Royal College of Surgeons of Edinburgh: http://www.rcsed.ac.uk
Royal College of Surgeons of England: http://www.rcseng.ac.uk
Royal Society of Medicine: http://www.rsm.ac.uk
The Society of Occupational Medicine: http://www.som.org.uk/

Working abroad

http://international.monster.com/workabroad/articles/health/
http://www.babelfish.altavista.com:
http://www.doctorsoftheworld.org/
http://www.fco.gov.uk/travel
http://www.holtmedical.com/workingabroad.htm
http://www.masta.org/
http://www.mediwork.info/

Medical resources

Agency for Healthcare Policy: http://www.ahcpr.gov/
Audit Commission: http://www.audit-commission.gov.uk
Best Medical Resources on the Web: http://www.priory.co.uk/othermed.htm
Centre for Evidence-based medicine: http://www.cebm.net/
Clinical Governance: http://www.clinicalgovernance.scot.nhs.uk/
Clinical Knowledge: http://www.cks.nhs.uk/home
Department of Health: http://www.doh.gov.uk
Doctors.net: http://www.doctors.net.uk/
General Medical Council: http://www.gmc-uk.org/
Health and Safety Executive (HSE): http://www.hse.gov.uk/hsehome.htm
King's Fund: http://www.kingsfund.org.uk/
Links to government websites: http://www.tagish.co.uk/tagish/links/
Medical Info Search: http://www.pavilion.co.uk/mednet/find_med.html
Medical Resource Database: http://www.hpdrc.fiu.edu/med.resource/
Medical Search Tools: http://wwnurse.com/medsearch.shtml
National Audit Office: http://www.nao.gov.uk/

National Network of Libraries of Medicine: http://nnlm.gov
NHS Centre for Evidence-Based Medicine: http://www.priory.co.uk/
othermed.htm
NHS Confederation: http://www.nhsconfed.co.uk/
NHS Direct Online: http://www.med.monash.edu.au/shcnlib/dehsj
NICE: http://www.nice.org.uk/
NPC – Audit handbook: http://www.npc.co.uk
PubMed (Medline): http://www.ncbi.nlm.nih.gov/PubMed/
SciTech Resources: http://www.scitechresources.gov
SHOW (Scottish Health on the Web): http://www.show.scot.nhs.uk/
Silver Platter Information: http://www.intelihealth.com/IH

Index

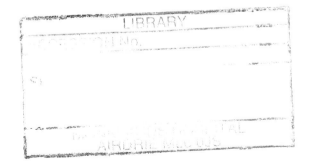